# NIGHTSHADE FREE

# PAIN FREE!

# MICHAEL FOWLER

Library of Congress cataloging ~ in ~ publication data

Nightshade Free Pain Free

Edited by: Jenny Bell

Cover photo: *Potato Flowers* by Keith Weller U.S. Dept. of Agriculture


ISBN: 978-0-9797728-0-1

# Potatoes are Poisonous

"Both the sprouts and green potatoes which grow at the soil surface have been responsible for fatal poisoning in humans" -Poisonous Plants of Pennsylvania

After the elimination of nightshade plants "...of the 52% rigidly on the diet, 94% reported complete or substantial relief of arthritis..."- Journal of Neurological and Orthopedic Medical Surgery (1993) 12:227-231

"Seventy-eight junior schoolboys in Great Britain became ill from solanine poisoning 7 to 9 hours after eating two small boiled peeled potatoes each (weight of potatoes not given) as part of their lunch, and 17 were admitted to hospital." (McMillan & Thompson)1979 .

"In 18 separate households in Scotland, 61 persons suffered typical 'solanine' poisoning soon to several hours after eating potatoes. Persons not eating potatoes were not ill. One 5-year-old died." (Harris & Cockburn, 1918).

"A three to four fold elevation of the potato glycoalkloids, solanine and chaconine (a teratogen), caused by a multiplicity of different environmental and physical conditions, **has killed more than 30 people and poisoned several thousand.** Because the symptoms of poisoning are very similar to bacterial food poisoning, many other thousands of poisonings are thought to go unremarked...5 cattle have died from eating green vine tomatoes containing tomatine. Consumption of 500g of potato at one meal will institute mild poisoning in sensitive people. The (long-term) chronic effects of solanine are unknown..."[1] [*]

---

[1] Anthony Trewavas of the Institute of Cell and Molecular Biology at the University of Edinburgh, UK.(Comment)", Chemistry and Industry, December 20, 2004.
[*] All emphasis is added by the author unless noted

"The common potato, *Solanum tuberosum*, contains toxic steroidal glycoalkaloids derived biosynthetically from cholesterol (Sharma & Salunkhe, 1989.... The potato glycoalkaloids have **not been evaluated previously** by the Joint FAO/WHO Expert Committee."

"Fifty-six German soldiers suffered typical 'solanine' poisoning after eating 1 to 1.5 kg cooked peeled potatoes containing 24 mg TGA/100 g (whole uncooked tubers contained 38 mg TGA/100g)."(Pfuhl,1899).

"In a recent (1983) poisoning associated with a school lunch programme, 61 of 109 school children and staff in Alberta, Canada, became ill, most within 5 minutes, after eating baked potato." (Anon, 1984).

"Cranial abnormalities have been observed in some teratogenicity[2] studies with laboratory animals, particularly with the hamster at levels of 165-200 mg glycoalkaloids/kg bw(*body weight*)/day." (Kuiper-Goodman and Nawrot)

"Two rhesus monkeys died 48 h after an i.p. injection of 40 mg/kg bw of total glycoalkaloids; one other died 2 h after having been dosed i.p. twice (24 h apart) with 20 mg solanine/kgbw"(Swinyard & Chaube, 1973).

Solanine found in potatoes is not only poisonous, it builds up over time. But, nobody ever told you any of this. Why?

---

[2] Teratogenicity: The production of monsters or misshapen organisms, ie. Birth Defects

# Dedication

This book is dedicated to a number of people, first. Karen who first informed me of solanine in potatoes. Next to Ricardo who helped me in dietary experiments, with his exquisite cooking. To all the people who encouraged me to write this book after I had given up, that would be you, Richard. The MWG. To the nurses, who showed so much love and kindness as a child in their work; you do really make a difference. To Jenny for her editing, comments and kindness. To my grandfather who taught me how to be brave. Lastly to my Mother and Father who suffered so much by having such a sickly son, for whom they did everything possible to cure.

# Foreword

Nothing in this book should constitute medical advice. This book has not been written as a manual on medicine, or for self-medication. The author is simply bringing to light many of the published reports that exist within the scientific community that have not received public attention.

As always, before any changes in diet, one should seek the advice of the medical doctor before proceeding. If you feel the suggestions contained within this book may be helpful for you, then consult your doctor and ask if a change of diet is permissible.

This book is a culmination of the author's research on the poisonous effects of nightshade plants in the human diet. It is to spark interest and research *to further understand* the ramifications of nightshades as a staple food in the human diet.

# Table of Contents

# Interactive Book

This is an interactive book. Meaning that the readers can respond to the content within this book. Because of recent technological advances, books do not need to remain static and unchanging. I sincerely ask that if you have comments, thoughts, information, or stories that you would like to share, please email them to me. It is my goal to improve this work as readers examine the contents.

michael@nightshadefree.com

# Introduction

You are very familiar with nightshade plants even if you do not recognize the term. Potatoes, tomatoes, eggplant, peppers, tobacco, jimson weed and more are all part of the nightshade family. They all contain poisons that attack the nervous system, the joints, the mind, and even cause cancer. Yes, it is true that the potato is the brother to the tobacco plant, and both contain the dreaded nicotine.

All nightshade plants contain nicotine that is a known source of cancer. A few spoonfuls of eggplant contain the same amount of nicotine as sitting in a closed room with a light-smoker for three hours. Recent studies have shown the nicotine seems to inhibit the body's ability to fight cancer, as it binds with the body's natural cancer fighting cells, preventing them from attacking cancer. Nightshade plants may be the leading cause of cancer in the world, and they are a staple food in most cultures. It is simply outrageous that studies on the long-term use of nightshades are not being done, especially, in light of the knowledge that cancer is a major epidemic and all nightshades contain nicotine. If my claim is true then simply removing nightshades from the diet will bring a great reduction in the incidence of cancer and many other diseases.

As we spend billions of dollars on research looking for cures to so many "incurable diseases" nightshades are completely ignored. It must be realized that what we have been doing for 50 years in research has failed to bring a cure. Therefore, our research must be called into question, and new approaches examined. It is fundamental and elementary consideration in investigative approaches. Please note I am not advocating any branch of medicine such as Chinese, or alternative, but issuing a wake up call to modern western medicine.

Nightshade plants contain more poisons than just nicotine; they also contain atropine, chaconine, tomatine, scopolamine, and more. Solanine is a cell disruptor; it can cause the lining of the cell wall to become inflamed leading to digestive problems. It is this action that caused me to do research on the poisons of nightshades. Some people are more sensitive to solanine than others are. Solanine caused me great intestinal distress, to the point of having diarrhea, severe abdominal cramps, and even bleeding from the intestines. All of this caused my digestive tract harm to the point that I became malnourished. At five years old, I weighed 37 lbs. I even had the "pot-belly" seen so often in starving African children. None of the doctors thought to eliminate nightshade plants from my diet. They did test me for allergies and I had none. Nightshades are one of the most allergy free foods available. I was not allergic to them, but was affected by the poison solanine.

By the time I was five the doctors with all of their tests had given up. My exhausted mother discovered I reacted well to chicken and rice and started to put on weight. So that is what I ate for a long time. However, nightshades continued to cause me distress. Sleepiness, weakness, muscle aches, abdominal cramps, and sometimes intestinal bleeding. It never went completely away even in adulthood. That is until I found out quite by accident about solanine in nightshades and eliminated them from my diet (*play heavenly music now*). I can now say that nightshade plants were the bane of my existence. This book is the results of my studies on nightshades in the human diet.

Of course, if my parents had been shown the reports in this book, on how nightshade can inflame the bowels, cause cramping and other digestive problems. It would have saved us thousands of dollars in tests, trips to the hospital, and endless heartache.

In spite of medical ignorance, I lived and went on to be a U.S. Marine, and was a member of the elite Force Recon unit. Nightshades continued to cause me harm and weakness even later in life, as joint problems and fatigue started to become constant. As time wore on bouts of severe of tiredness and abdominal cramps became chronic. It often interfered with my work, as after lunch I would be nearly unable to think or stay awake.

On several occasions, I went to the emergency room thinking I was suffering from food poisoning. One time, my heart started to beat erratically, so they performed a complete E.K.G on me from head to toe. They said I might have been the healthiest person they had ever tested. My resting heartbeat after a few hours was 42 beats per minute, and I was excited, (that was a long time ago). By the time I had arrived at the emergency room the toxic effects were dissipating, and I was recovering. Needless, to say I felt like a fool at the time. E.R. visits are not cheap.

It is because of these experiences with nightshades that I figure there might be some other sickly little boys and girls out there who do not want to grow up malnourished, with intestinal disorders. Perhaps you might not benefit from this information, but I bet you know someone who can, and it is our duty to learn and inform those around us about the various dangers in life.

Nightshades are injuring more than just me. Many others are suffering from the poisons in these plants and have no idea. These poisons are causing everything from cramps to cancer, arthritis to migraines, and more.

All nightshades contain small amounts of several neurotoxins. Some nightshades, such as mandrake, contain large amounts of these neurotoxins. If one would ever eat a mandrake plant instead of a potato, the term nightshade would become abundantly clear; the Greek term nightshade means death. These plants were used for just such purposes in the Middle Ages, and earlier, for poisoning.

Quite a bit of hay has been made about so many foods being bad for us. White flour, deep-fried foods, sugar, the list is quite long, and now I am telling you that nightshade plants are bad for you too! "*No! You can't take away my potatoes or tomatoes, I love them!*" you might protest. Well, I like them too. Many people like tobacco, but it is bad for you. However, I do want you to hear this point. Nightshades are the ONLY foods we eat that as a staple contain neurotoxins. You can process sugar, your body loves sugar, the problem with sugar is not that it is toxic; the problem is that people eat too much of it. White flour is not bad for you, but a steady diet of it is. The big difference is all other foods can be processed by your digestive system. Nightshades are good for you except for the neurotoxins that cannot be extracted from them easily, and cooking does **not** noticeably affect them. When we eat nightshades, we are receiving a daily dose of drugs that do not leave the body quickly, and can cause lots of damage.

We are all familiar with the effects of tobacco. We also know about carcinogens it contains. Few of us understand that tobacco and potato come from the same family, the nightshades. Most people understand that smoking once in awhile does not have any harmful effects on the human being. If one were to smoke, say once a month, it would be of no concern, with the exception of its potential addictive qualities.

The same holds true with any other member of the nightshade family. Small use is almost of no effect for most people. Sure, you may want to put a little dash of Paprika (a nightshade) on some cottage cheese; well, go ahead, but do not make potatoes a staple food. Long-term use can lead to dramatic disabilities. For some people even small use can have severe results.

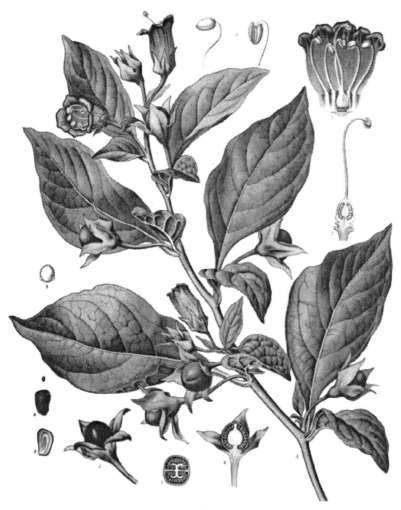

Atropa belladonna L.

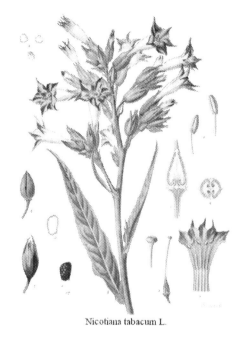

*Nicotiana tabacum L.*

First things first, it is necessary to explain exactly what are nightshade plants. It has been my experience that many people are unsure about nightshade botany. The following pages will be an explanation of the plants in this family.

*Image: Tobacco Plant*

The nightshade family is called <u>Solanaceae</u> in Latin, so I will refer to the *Solanaceae* family as *nightshades*, since we speak English. Often people have asked me, "is lettuce a nightshade?" or "sweet potatoes?", "what about wheat?", and I am pleased to inform them that, none of those are members of the nightshade family. The following is an overview of nightshade plants. Of the foods we *eat*, only the following are nightshades and no others:

Potatoes, tomatoes, most peppers, and eggplant.

Before potatoes were introduced as a food, they were understood by the peasant class as poisonous. It was easy for them to tell because the flowers of Deadly Nightshade and potatoes are nearly the same. We classify plants by external appearance. When the same features are seen in two kinds of plants, then they are of the same family. Solanum is a large, variable genus of annual plants and perennial plants, forbs, vines, sub-shrubs, shrubs, and small trees. They often have attractive fruit and flowers.

**The flowers** have five petals, normally fused, start in a funnel shape and progress wider until the petal tips point backwards from the center. Petals are often yellow, white, or blue and have a five-pointed star.

**The leaves** are often have a hairy or clammy surface. Often the first leaves will have purple undersides.

**The fruit** of nightshades are berries, such as the tomato, or a *dehiscent* which becomes dry and breaks open releasing seeds capsule as seen in the Mandrake. Fruit starts green and turns dark purple to black or red

**The seeds** are small, round and flat, approximately 2-4mm in diameter. As seen in the common tomato.

**The stamens** the center cone, are normally four parts but are sometimes eight. Generally they are yellow in color and cone shaped.

**Flowers of Nightshades:**

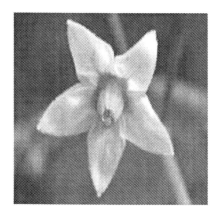

Deadly Nightshade[1]

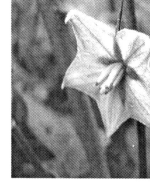

Eggplant

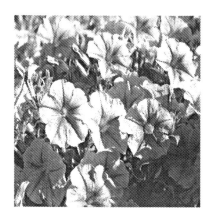

Pink Petunias

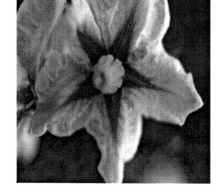

Potato

# Fruit of Nightshades

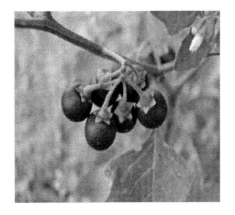

Deadly Nightshade[3]

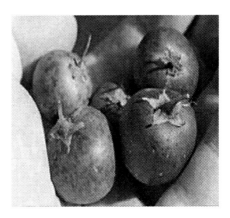

Potato fruit[4]

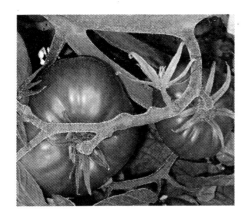

Tomato

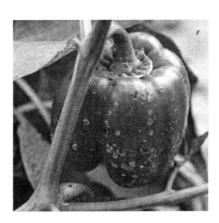

Bell Pepper[5]

---

[3] Oregon State University
[4] Dr. David Midgley
[5] Univeristy of Massachusetts, Amherst

# Scientific classification of Nightshades

| Kingdom: | Plantae |
|---|---|
| Division: | Magnoliophyta |
| Class: | Magnoliopsida |
| Subclass: | Asteridae |
| Order: | Solanales |
| Family: | Solanaceae |

## Genra

- S. aculeastrum - Sodaapple nightshade
- S. adscendens - Sonoita nightshade
- S. aethiopicum - Ethiopian nightshade or nakati
- S. americanum - Purple or glossy nightshade; American black nightshade; Poroporo
- S. arcanum
- S. aviculare - Poroporo
- S. bahamense - Bahama nightshade
- S. bulbocastanum - Ornamental nightshade
- S. burbankii - Wonderberry
- S. campechiense - Redberry nightshade
- S. capsicastrum - False Jerusalem cherry
- **S. capsicum - Chile peppers**
- S. capsicoides - Cockroach berry
- S. cardiophyllum - Heartleaf nightshade
- S. carolinense - Apple of Sodom, Horsenettle
- S. centrale - Australian desert raisin
- S. chenopodioides - Goosefoot nightshade
- S. citrullifolium - Watermelon nightshade
- S. clokeyi - Clokey's nightshade
- S. commersonii - Commerson's nightshade
- S. conocarpum - Marron bacoba
- S. davisensen - Davis horsenettle
- S. demissum - Dwarf wild potato
- S. dimidiatum - Torrey's nightshade
- S. diphyllum - Twinleaf nightshade
- S. donianum - Mullein nightshade
- S. douglasii - Greenspot nightshade
- S. drymophilum - Erubia
- S. dulcamara - Bittersweet
- S. elaeagnifolium - Silverleaf nightshade
- S. ellipticum - Potato bush

- S. erianthum - Mullein nightshade, Potato tree
- S. fendleri - Fendler's horsenettle
- S. ferox - Hairy-fruited eggplant, Thai hairy-fruited eggplant
- S. furcatum - Forked nightshade
- S. gayanum - Chilean nightshade
- S. gilo - Scarlet Eggplant, Gilo (Brazilian jiló)
- S. glacum -
- S. glaucophyllum - Waxyleaf nightshade
- S. gracilius - Slender nightshade
- S. heterodoxum - Melon-leaf nightshade
- S. hindsianum - Hinds' nightshade
- S. hyporhodium - synonym of S. sessiliflorum
- S. imcompletum -
- S. incanum -
- S. incompletum - Popolo ku mai
- S. interius -
- S. jamaicense - Jamaican nightshade
- S. jamesii - Wild potato
- S. jasminoides - Jasmine nightshade
- S. khasianum - Indian nightshade
- S. lanceifolium - Lanceleaf nightshade
- S. lanceolatum - Orangeberry nightshade
- S. leptosepalum - Tigna potato
- S. linnaeanum - Apple of Sodom (Hawaii)
- S. lumholtzianum - Sonoran nightshade
- S. lycocarpum - Wolf Apple
- **S. lycopersicum - Tomato**
- S. macrocarpon -
- S. marginatum - White-margined nightshade
- S. mauritianum - Earleaf nightshade
- S. melanocerasum - Garden huckleberry
- **S. melongena - Eggplant**
- S. mucronatum - Pepino
- S. muricatum - Pepino
- S. nelsonii - Nelson's horsenettle
- S. nigrescens - Divine nightshade
- S. nigrum - Black or blackberry nightshade
- S. nudum - Forest nightshade
- S. parishii - Parish's nightshade
- S. pericifolium
- S. persicifolium - Berengena de playa
- S. peruvianum - Peruvian nightshade
- S. phureja -
- S. physalifolium - Hairy nightshade
- S. pimpinellifolium - Currant tomato
- S. pinnatisectum - Tansyleaf nightshade
- S. polygamum - Cakalaka berry
- S. pseudogracile - Glowing nightshade
- S. ptycanthum - Eastern black nightshade

- S. pyrifolium -
- S. quitoense - Naranjilla
- S. racemosum - Canker berry
- S. riedlei - Riedle's nightshade
- S. robustum - Shrubby nightshade
- S. rostratum - Texas thistle
- S. rugosum - Tabacon aspero
- S. sandwicense - Hawaii horsenettle
- S. sarrachoides - Green nightshade
- S. seaforthianum - Brazilian nightshade
- S. sessiliflorum - Cocona
- S. sisymbriifolium - Sticky nightshade
- S. surattense -
- S. tampicense - Wetland nightshade
- S. tenuilobatum - San Diego nightshade
- S. tenuipes - Fancy nightshade
- S. torvum - Devil's fig
- S. triflorum Nutt. - Cutleaf nightshade
- S. triquetrum - Texas nightshade
- **S. tuberosum - Potato**
- S. umbelliferum - Bluewitch nightshade
- S. viarum - Tropical soda apple
- S. villosum - Hairy nightshade
- S. viride - Green nightshade cv. form from Fiji: S. anthropophagorum
- S. wallacei - Wallace's nightshade, Catalina Nightshade
- S. wendlandii - Giant potatocreeper
- S. woodburyi - Woodbury's nightshade
- S. xanthi
- S. xanti - Purple nightshade

*Note: edible in bold*

## Culinary Concerns (nightshade substitutes)

Before warning you of the dangers of nightshades, I want to tell you about other foods that you can eat instead. Our worst enemy is our desires–they far outweigh our good sense. Thus, let us examine nightshade substitutes beforehand. It makes the rest of the book easier to stomach (I had to say that.) Just because you may wish to eliminate nightshades from your diet, it does not mean you cannot enjoy good food. In fact, night-shades have so dominated cooking that many other great foods have been pushed aside needlessly, so here are some replacement ideas.

**Potatoes:** They taste awful. They really do, few people like them without toppings such as butter.

*"None for me. I appreciate the potato only as a protection against famine; except for that, I know of nothing more eminently tasteless."*
- Anthelme Brillat-Savarin (1755-1826), French politician and writer on gastronomy

Try eating a plain potato (no salt, no butter, no good); you will not like it. Butter makes everything taste better, so does bacon. We like the toppings we put on potatoes, not the potatoes themselves.
Sweet potatoes are twice as good for you as potatoes, and taste good without toppings. Just replace potatoes with sweet potatoes; they are much better for you.

### Sweet potatoes

*Sweet potato*

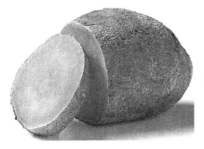

In 2007 Dr. Jon Allen, professor of food science, College of Agriculture and Life Sciences, North Carolina State University, released a report that sweet potatoes have a low gylcemic index(GI) and may even aid reducing diabetes.[6]

In 1992 the *Center for Science in the Public Interest* compared the nutritional value of sweet potatoes to all other table vegetables. Considering fiber content, complex carbohydrates, protein, vitamins A and C, iron, and calcium, the sweet potato ranked highest in nutritional value. According to these criteria, sweet potatoes earned 184 points, 100 points over the next on the list, the common potato. (NCSPC) [7]

**Nutrition information per serving of one medium sweet potato:**

| | |
|---|---|
| Calories | 130 |
| Calories from fat | 0.39 g |
| Protein | 2.15 g |
| Carbohydrate | 31.56 g |
| Dietary Fiber | 3.9 g |
| Sodium | 16.9 mg |
| Potassium | 265.2 mg |
| Calcium | 28.6 mg |
| Folate | 18.2 mcg |
| Vitamin C | 29.51 mg |
| Vitamin A | 26081.9 IU |

Source: National Agricultural Library (NAL), part of the Agricultural Research Service of the US Department of Agriculture.

Are yams and sweet potatoes (I. batatas), same thing? No. Some folks think sweet potatoes are yams (Dioscorea batatas), which are not from the same family, but are similar in appearance. Yams are not grown in the continental U.S.–sweet potatoes are. Neither yams nor sweet potatoes are part of the nightshade family and are wonderful to eat. According to 2004 FAO statistics, world production of sweet potatoes is 127,000,000 tons. North Carolina, the leading U.S. state in sweet potato production, currently provides 40% of the annual U.S. production of sweet potatoes.

---

[6] NC State University researchers reveal sweet potato as weapon against diabetes by Suzanne Stanard, Department of Communications, NC State University
[7] Louisiana Sweet Potato Commission, Louisiana Department of Agriculture and Forestry, http://www.sweetpotato.org/

*Tongan farmer showing off his prize (true) yams, (Dioscorea batatas) Photo by* James Foster 1986

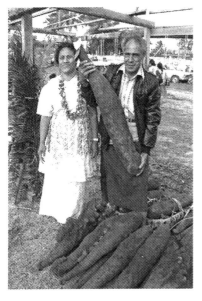

**Pastas:** It might be hard to imagine a time when Italian cooking was without tomato-based sauces, but it is true! They did not exist until the 19th century. Before that, cheese, olive oils, and spices ruled the flavors of pasta. Pasta with olive oil, garlic and cheese is a sure delight. Think of creamy alfredo sauce on your pasta dishes. Now the that local pizzerias are kind enough to make delicious nightshade free sauces, called white sauces, tomato sauce is no longer necessary.

Ranch dressings are a great substitute for tomatoes. Ranch can be used on chicken wings, burgers, and more. Many fast-food chains are now using ranch dressings instead of ketchup or Bar-B-Q sauces. Before ketchup existed, mustards and mayonnaise sauced the sandwiches and meats. Onion rings instead of fries, take care of that burger and coke combo.

**Peppers, Peppers, and Peppercorns, who is who?**

There is so much confusion with peppers, it seemed best to include what is and is not a nightshade pepper.

Nightshades peppers are the following: bell, banana, wax, chili, Thai, red, green, datil, habanero, etc.

# The following peppers are *NOT* nightshade peppers:

### Black, White, and Green pepper

The berries are cooked briefly in hot water, both to clean them and to prepare them for drying. The berries are dried in the sun or by machine for several days, during which the fruit around the seed shrinks and darkens into a thin, wrinkled black layer. Once dried, the fruits are called black peppercorns.

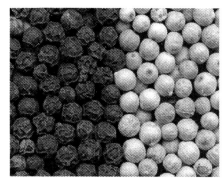

White pepper consists of the seed only, with the fruit removed. Use white pepper when black pepper would disturb the color of the food, such as white colored dishes, i.e. white fish. Green pepper, like black, is made from the unripe berries.

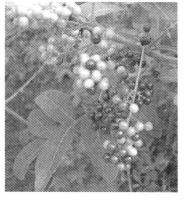

**Brazilian Pepper** (Schinus terebinthifolius; also known as Aroeira, Florida holly, and Christmas berry) is a sprawling shrub or small tree (7-10 m tall).

It is native to subtropical and tropical South America, in southeastern Brazil, northern Argentina and Paraguay. Not a nightshade, can be somewhat spicy, and can be toxic.

*Image: Schinus terebinthifolius, Brazilian Pepper, courtesy of U.S.G.S. (the dark berries are bright red in color).*

**Sichuan pepper (or Szechuan pepper)** is the outer pod of the tiny fruit of a number of species in the genus Zanthoxylum widely grown and consumed in Asia as a spice. It is not related to black pepper or to nightshade peppers and is popular in the cuisine of Sichuan, China, from which it takes its name.

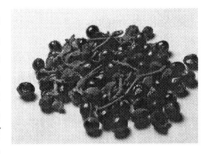

Sichuan pepper has a unique aroma and flavor that is not hot or pungent like black or white pepper, or chili peppers, but has slight lemony overtones and creates in the mouth a kind of tingly numbness[8] that prepares the palette for hot spices.

**Tasmannia** is a genus of woody, evergreen flowering plants of the family Winteraceae. The species of Tasmannia are native to Australia, New Guinea, Celebes, Borneo, and Philippines. Introduced into cultivation in Cornwall, U.K., it became the "Cornish pepperleaf" associated with Cornish cuisine.

**Long pepper** (Piper longum), sometimes called Indonesian Long Pepper, is a flowering vine in the family Piperaceae, cultivated for its fruit, which is usually dried and used as a spice and seasoning. Long pepper is a close relative of the black pepper plant, and has a similar, though generally hotter taste.

### The secrets of pepper cooking:

When black pepper is added during cooking the heat dulls the favor of the pepper; it is better to add it at the end. The exception is when you want lots of heat, and do not want lots of pepper flavor.

If the meal is cooked with Szechuan pepper and enough freshly ground black pepper is added, it can increase the heat to the point of

---

[8] caused by its 3% of hydroxy-alpha-sanshool

making the toughest of tongues want water. If you like heat, then Szechuan pepper is your friend, as it really allows the heat to come on strong.

According to George Mateljan, black pepper aids digestion by stimulating the taste buds in a way that alerts the stomach to produce acid, (hydrochloric acid); this greatly aids in improving the digestion of proteins and carbohydrates. When this production of acid is low, the components of food cannot be unlocked and the intestines will not be able to digest the food; this leads to burping and heartburn, then gas and diarrhea. Nightshades in the diet decrease the body's ability to digest food as they deaden the nerves in the digestive tract.

Another study on *piperine*, found in black pepper, showed an increase of digestive bioavailability when black pepper was introduced.[9] It increased the ability of normally poorly absorbed nutrients by the intestine and liver up to 2000%.[10]

---

[9] Effects of piperine, the pungent component of black pepper, at the human vanilloid receptor (TRPV1).
FN McNamara, A Randall, MJ Gunthorpe, GI-CEDD, GlaxoSmithKline, New Fronteirs Science Park, Third Avenue, Harlow, Essex CM19 5AW.
[10] Influence of piperine on pharmacokinetics of curcumin in aminal and human vlunteers, Shoba, et el. Department of Pharmacolgy, St. John's Medical College, Bangalore, India, Panta Medica 1998, 64, p. 353-356.

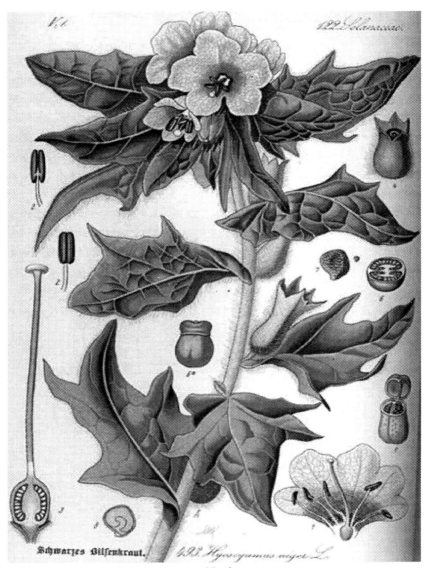

Henbane

*Hemlock is a vegetable, just as vulture's flesh is flesh yet no one in his senses would eat henbane nor dog's flesh unless he were in very great straits.*
*-St. Basil the Great*

# Part I: History of Nightshades

*The berries of the belladonna or deadly nightshade, produce, when eaten, a furious madness, followed by sleep, which lasts for twenty-four hours. Such drugs as produce mental stupefaction, without impairing the physical powers, may have given rise to the accounts of men being transformed into brutes, so frequent in what are denominated the fabulous writers, while the evanescent but exquisite joys of an opposite description, an anticipation of what implicit obedience would ensure them for ever, produced blind, furious, devoted adherents to any philosophical speculator, who would venture to try so desperate an experiment.*

*– Thaumaturgia by An Oxonian, 1835*

For centuries nightshade plants were known to be poisonous, from long before the time of Christ, they were used to poison, harm and seduce. It is nothing new, that someone should say nightshades are poisonous. We believe the potatoes a nightshade are a healthy food, but we forget that inside are small amounts of vicious poison, that build up in our system over time.

There is a mythos that all foods we eat are healthy until someone proves that is unhealthy; however, we know differently. It took years to discover the connection between smoking and lung cancer, almost 300 years to be exact. We cannot say that all of the necessary research about cancer and other diseases has been performed as long as those diseases are still with us. There is nothing wrong with being observant and learning new information about the foods we eat.

Nightshades may or may not be a source of health problems for you, but they certainly are for some. The health effects of nightshades should be known by all people, just as smoking is, so they can make a determination as to whether or not they wish to eat something that contains toxins.

A great number of people are completely unaware that if potatoes show any green at all, that the whole potato must be thrown out. Some people suspect they can cut out the green and use the rest of the potato. This is in error, as the solanine spreads throughout the potato evenly, especially in the skin. The green color (from chlorophyll) alerts us to the fact that this potato has been exposed to light. It is this exposure to light that will dramatically increase the solanine content throughout the potato. It is not the green part that is rotten or bad; it is the increase in Solanine within that makes green potatoes poisonous.

The poison solanine can even increase in the dark at 20 percent of the rate in the light. Under common retail displays, the amount of solanine can increase to exceed the safe limits by nine times within 24 hours. This increase in solanine is not always accompanied with greening of the skin. Bruising or being grown in cold climates will also increase solanine.

To prevent exposure to light potatoes were sold in burlap bags. Now they are displayed out in the open in supermarkets, or in transparent plastic bags that allow light.

## The Three Hags

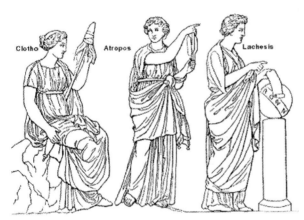

I have included the history of nightshades, because people often have questions as to how these foods were introduced. Atropa Belladonna is the scientific name for Deadly Nightshade. The term nightshade means to bring down the shade of death, to end the light of life.

Atropos is the Greek word for one of the three Greek fates, who were timeless old hags in Greek mythology, the three daughters of Zeus and Themis. These three sisters would control the thread of life the first was Clotho, who would spin the thread of life; the second was Lachesis, who would determine the length of life or yarn, as the case may be. The last and most dreaded was Atropos, who cut the thread of life; she was the bringer of death. The ancient Greeks believed that these three controlled the destiny of your life. These three even wove good and evil into your thread of life. They were so powerful that even the gods themselves were subject to their designs.

Now, for the other half of the name: Belladonna. It is an Italian or Latin word: *Bella* means beautiful, and *donna* means lady. It received this name long ago, when young women would pluck the berries from the atropine belladonna plant, and then squeeze them, allowing the drops to fall into their eyes. The juice of the berry would cause the pupils to dilate. This would give these young girls a wide-eyed innocent look that was all the fashion at the time. One could see how it adopted the name belladonna.[11] It fell out of fashion when it was found that atropine could be adsorbed into the bloodstream via the eye, and atropine poisoning would ensue. Often, this would result in death.

## Pagan Madness

This poisonous fruit had other uses as well, some of them quite un-savory. It was mixed into wine as an hallucinogenic by the phallus-worshiping cult of the god Bacchus. This cult was so out of control that it was banned by the Romans, who were pagan at that time, as a menace to society itself. The image below on the cult of Bacchus even had to be edited, for decency's sake, in order to be included in this book. Shown below is a prominent Roman citizen being carried back home after a night of scandalous indecency.[12]

---

[11] Fackelmann, Kathy A.. "Food, drug, or poison? (toxic plants used by tribal cultures as food or medicine) (Cover Story)", Science News, May 15, 1993.
[12] "CABINET SECRET" by Colonel Fanin.(Stanislas Marie César Famin, b. 1799 d. 1853)

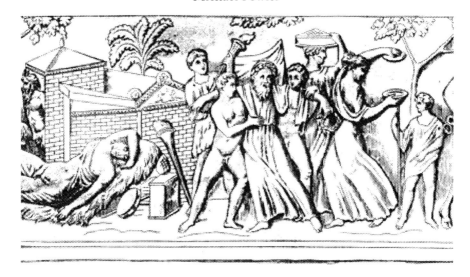

*The cult of Bacchus*

Some of the reports of the time include mass rapes of men and women, running wild in the streets, tearing apart animals and eating them raw. In fact, it is scopolamine from the nightshade plants that is now used in the nefarious "date rape" drug[13]. This is considered a very dangerous drug, as it blocks the mind's ability to create memories. Does a diet of nightshades, which contain scopolamine, affect our students' ability to learn?

Scopolamine (also known as Hyoscine) can be found in a variety of non-prescription sedatives, such as *Sominex*. It is similar to the neurotransmitter acetylcholine; it acts by interfering with the transmission of nerve impulses by acetylcholine in the parasympathetic nervous system. Typical symptoms of exposure include dilated pupils, rapid heartbeat, and drying of the skin, mouth, and respiratory passages.

Because scopolamine depresses the central nervous system, it is used as a sedative prior to anesthesia, but can also be used to treat various

---

[13] Published by: Richters, Canada's Herb Specialists Goodwood, Ontario L0C 1A0, Canada Editor: Conrad Richter

disorders characterized by restlessness and agitation, such as delirium tremens, psychosis, manias, and Parkinson's disease.

Young women in Central America who have been given this drug at parties, by slipping it into their drinks, have become so compliant that they will give up their babies, and be used as prostitutes. Unofficial estimates indicate that there are approximately 50,000 scopolamine incidents in Colombia per year.[14] In Bogota, the greater number of victims are men who appear wealthy, and are approached by attractive young women. The "lady's" friends then mug these drugged men. Overdoes will cause respiratory failure, which results in death.

> BOGOTA, Colombia (Reuters) - The last thing Andrea Fernandez recalls before being drugged is holding her newborn baby on a Bogota city bus.
>
> Police found her three days later, muttering to herself and wandering topless along the median strip of a busy highway. Her face was badly beaten and her son was gone.
>
> Fernandez is just one of hundreds of victims every month who, according to Colombian hospitals, are temporarily turned into zombies by a home-grown drug called scopolamine which has been embraced by thieves and rapists.
>
> "When I woke up in the hospital, I asked for my baby and nobody said anything. They just looked at me," Fernandez said, weeping. Police believe her son Diego was taken by a gang which traffics in infants.
>
> Colorless, odorless and tasteless, scopolamine is slipped into drinks and sprinkled onto food. Victims become so docile that they have been known to help thieves rob their homes and empty their bank accounts. Women have been drugged repeatedly over days and gang-raped or rented out as prostitutes.[15]

Entire weeks of abuse do not exist in their minds because the memories were never created nor installed in the mind. It is also the base for many wonderful drugs that are used in preventing motion sickness. The chemical formula for scopolamine is $C_{17}H_{21}NO_4$. The chemical formula for cocaine is the same $C_{17}H_{21}NO_4$. The two compounds have the same

---

[14] Colombia 2007 Crime & Safety Report; Overseas Security Advisory Council; Bureau of Diplomatic Security; U.S. Department of State • Washington, D.C.
[15] *Drug Turns Crime Victims Into Zombies*, By Phil Stewart

molecular formula but different structural formulas, thereby accounting for the different effects.

In 1963, the US Supreme Court said in Townsend v. Sain, 372 U.S. 293, that "serum-induced confession" was in effect a form of torture and the practice was ruled unconstitutional.

> "*It is at least generally recognized that the administration of sufficient doses of scopolamine will break down the will. ...The early literature on the subject designated scopolamine as a "truth serum." It was thought to produce true confessions by criminal suspects.*"[16] ....However, whether scopolamine produces true confessions or false confessions, it in fact caused Townsend to make statements, those statements were constitutionally inadmissible.[17]

The Oracle of Delphi, in Greece, was considered the greatest center of prophecy in the world. The activities that were performed at this place were so profane that they cannot be retold in this book. However, it was

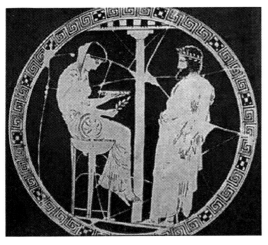

the Atropine Belladonna, that again was mixed into wine and the mandrakes that were smeared over the bodies of the visitors, that sent them into frenzies of madness. This atropine poisoning causes many rabies-like symptoms, such as frothing at the mouth.

Poisoning has long been a much feared and dreaded tool of the wicked.

---

[16] E. g., House, *Why Truth Serum Should be Made Legal*, 42 Medico-Legal Journal 138 (1925). And as recently as 1940 Dean Wigmore suggested that scopolamine might be useful in criminal interrogation. 3 Wigmore on Evidence (3d ed. 1940) § 998, at 642.

[17] *Interrogation under Drug Influence. The So-Called "Truth Serum" Technique*
C. W. Muehlberger, The Journal of Criminal Law, Criminology, and Police Science, Vol. 42, No. 4 (Nov. - Dec., 1951), pp. 513-528

The terrible problem with poisonings were that at first it could be hard to distinguish from a common illness, and second is that little could be done. A popular example is was nightshade Henbane. I mention it here for two reasons: how it can be administered, via the ear, and two, was called "leprous"; that will be important later on in this text. It was mentioned by Shakespeare when the ghost (Hamlet's father) from *Hamlet* (I,5, 69-70) revealed how he was killed to young Hamlet by having the nightshade henbane poured into his ear:[18]

Hamlet: *Murder!*

Ghost: *Murder most foul, as in the best it is;*
*But this most foul, strange, and unnatural.....*
　　*Sleeping within my orchard*
　　*My custom always of the afternoon*
　　*Upon my safe and secure hour thy uncle stole*
　　*With juice of cursed hebona [henbane] in a vial*
　　*And in the porches of my ears did pour*
　　*The leprous distillment whose effect*
　　*Holds such an enmity with blood of man*
　　*That swift as quicksilver it courses through*
　　*The natural gates and alleys of the body.*

In those days there were no laboratories to analyze the poisons so as to treat it properly, not that it would have done much good. The doctors had to be found, by members of the family whether on foot or horseback; no cell phones, no "life-flight," and few cures. The only solution then was to purge the victim, and give them something to coat the linings of the stomach, such as milk or butter. Sometimes the cures were worse than the poison; often "quicksilver" (mercury) was recommended as a treatment. If the poison did not kill you, the mercury would.

Atropine is used by anesthesiologists to control mucus development during general anesthesia, so patients will not suffocate; it dries out

---

[18] *Shakespeare and Medicine, or The Medical and Surgical Knowledge of William Shakespeare.* by John William Wainwright

the membranes. It is also used in ophthalmology to expand the pupil so the doctor may examine the eyes.

## Nightshades in the Bible

Another nightshade is the mandrake mentioned in the Bible in Genesis. When the Bible mentions a food or an animal, it names a type as a whole, not a particular species. What I mean by this is that the Bible refers to family types, so mandrakes would refer to all nightshades in general. However, at that time I am sure it meant mandrake specifically, as potatoes were only found in Central America. [19] Mandrake in Hebrew is "duday", meaning "love plant" (aphrodisiac)[20]. It was believed by Asian cultures to ensure conception. Most interpreters hold *Mandragora officinarum* to be the plant intended in Genesis 30:14 (love-philtre), and Song of Solomon 7:13 (smell of the mandrakes). Many of the books of the occult also mention the mandrake as an aphrodisiac, "*The natural mandragore ... It is slightly narcotic, and an aphrodisiacal virtue was ascribed to it by the ancients, who represented it as being sought by Thessalian sorcerers for the composition of philters(love potions).*"[21]

Genesis 30:14-16 *And Reuben went in the days of wheat harvest, and found mandrakes in the field, and brought them unto his mother Leah. Then Rachel said to Leah, "Give me, I pray thee, of thy son's mandrakes." And she said unto her, "Is it a small matter that thou hast taken my husband? and wouldest thou take away my son's mandrakes also?" And Rachel said, "Therefore he shall lie with thee tonight for thy son's mandrakes." And Jacob came out of the field in the evening, and Leah went out to meet him, and said, "Thou must come in unto me; for surely I have hired thee with my son's mandrakes." And he lay with her that night.* [22]

---

[19] Agricultural Research Service botanist David M. Spooner "*New clues to origin of potatoes.*", M2 Presswire, March 18, 2005.

[20] *Strong's exhaustive concordance* by James Strong,1890 From H1731; a boiler or basket; also the mandrake (as aphrodisiac): - basket, mandrake.

[21] Chapter XVI, *Witchcraft and Spells: Transcendental Magic its Doctrine and Ritual* by Eliphas Levi. A Complete Translation of Dogme et Rituel de la Haute Magie by Arthur Edward Waite. 1896

[22] King James version

Song of Solomon 7:13 *The mandrakes give a smell, and at our gates are all manner of pleasant fruits, new and old, which I have laid up for thee, O my beloved.* [23]

The Bible speaks of mandrakes, which are part of the nightshade family. More aptly, it speaks of them growing with wheat. This is of interest as this is the exact problem mentioned by the Apostles in the Gospels, (Matt. 13:25) *"Lord, we see tares growing among the wheat."* Tares (*Lolium temulentum*) are a grass with poisonous seeds, and not part of the nightshade family. Peasants were sometimes poisoned with tares when they failed to follow the Biblical injunction to separate them from the grain. The same would be true of nightshades growing in the fields. To this day ranchers must be wary of nightshades growing in cattle feeds.

Its ability to provoke lust was also noted by William Salmon, in The Family Dictionary, or Household Companion, 1695: They Astringe, are moderately Diuretic, Stomatic, Chylisic, Analeptic, and Spermatogenetic. They nourish the whole body, restore in consumptions, and provoke lust... as common food: they increase seed and provoke lust, causing fruitfulness in both sexes: and stop all sorts of fluxes of the belly.

## Witchcraft and Nightshades

### Mandrake

Mandrakes were highly feared; it was thought that they contained an evil spirit which would attack and kill the one who removed it from the ground. It was a crime of witchcraft punishable by death even to have a mandrake in one's home.

They found their way into the popular children's books by J. K. Rowling. Mandrake is used to revive people who have been petrified in Harry Potter and the Chamber of Secrets.

---

[23] King James version

From Chapter 6:

*"Now, who can tell me the properties of the Mandrake?"...*

*"Mandrake or Mandragora is a powerful restorative," said Hermione, sounding as usual as though she had swallowed the textbook. "It is used to return people who have been transfigured or cursed, to their original state."*

*"Excellent. Ten points to Gryffindor," said Professor Sprout. "The Mandrake forms an essential part of most antidotes. It is also, however, dangerous. Who can tell me why?"*

*Hermione's hand narrowly missed Harry's glasses as it shot up again. "The cry of the Mandrake is fatal to anyone who hears it," she said promptly.*

*"Precisely. Take another ten points," said Professor Sprout.*

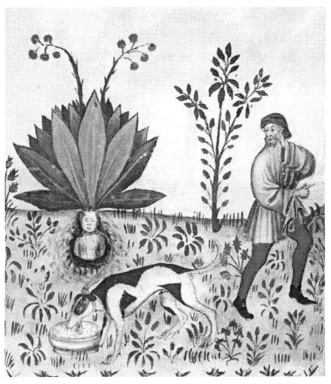

*Figure 1: Medieval drawing of harvesting a Mandrake (The dog is tied to the Mandrake plant)*

*"A furrow must be dug around the root until its lower part is exposed, then a dog is tied to it, after which the person tying the dog must get away. The dog then endeavours to follow him, and so easily pulls up the root, but dies suddenly instead of his master. After this the root can be handled without fear."* [24]

In the illustration, the dog (who had not been fed for a number of days) is given food to occupy it until the harvester (pointing to his own direction of travel and with his other hand upon his cheek denoting lament for the dog) gets far enough away to avoid the plant's vengeance. All of this is so strange that I think it was a rumor produced by "witches" to prevent peasants from killing the rare and valuable mandrake plants. How many times would you have a dog pull this plant from the ground, and not find him dead, before you would realize that fable was false?

Certainly one could imagine the shock when the first brave fellow, in front of everyone, yanked one from the ground and nothing happened. Of course, he had probably tested this a time or two with a dog in the midst of the night, beforehand, just to be sure. Also, note the bright red fruit of the mandrake showing relation to the tomato; even the array of the fruits is the same. One also wonders at the horribly bad advice contained in the Harry Potter book about them being an antidote; they are only an antidote for life or sanity.

Harvesters were also told to plug their ears with wax to avoid hearing the mandrake's cry when it was pulled from the ground. To hear its cry was thought to be fatal.

*"Shrieks like mandrakes' torn out of the earth."*
Shakespeare: Romeo and Juliet, iv. m3.

*"Would curses kill, as doth the mandrake's groan"*
King Henry VI Part 2 Act 3. Scene II

In other accounts of witches: the witch washed the root in wine and wrapped it in silk and velvet. She then fed it with sacramental wafers stolen from a church during communion.

---

[24] from the late 14th century manuscript herbal Theatrum Sanitatis (f. LXXIII, Ms. 4182). Some sources credit Josephus (c. 37 AD/CE Jerusalem – c. 100)

In the Extract from Chapter XVI, of *Witchcraft and Spells: Transcendental Magic its Doctrine and Ritual* by Eliphas Levi. (A Complete Translation of Dogma et Ritual de la Haute Maggie by Arthur Edward Waite. 1896) the following account of mandrakes is given:

*"... The natural mandragore is a filamentous root which, more or less, presents as a whole either the figure of a man, or that of the virile members. It is slightly narcotic, and an aphrodisiacal virtue was ascribed to it by the ancients, who represented it as being sought by Thessalian sorcerers for the composition of philtres[25]. Is this root the umbilical vestige of our terrestrial origin? We dare not seriously affirm it, but all the same it is certain that man came out of the slime of the earth, and his first appearance must have been in the form of a rough sketch.*

Concoctions that used nightshades were used to induce sleep. A typical one from 12th-15th century English manuscripts includes both mandrake and henbane. The following is for a sedative strong enough to numb a person for surgery.

*The above is English*

*"How to make a drink that men call dwale to make a man sleep whilst men cut him: take three spoonfuls of the gall [bile] of a barrow swine [boar] for a man, and for a woman of a gilt [sow], three spoonfuls of*

---

[25] Philtres: Philo is greek for love, phitres are love plants.

*hemlock juice, three spoonfuls of wild neep [bryony]* (mandrake)*, three spoonfuls of lettuce, three spoonfuls of pape [opium], three spoonfuls of henbane, and three spoonfuls of eysyl [vinegar], and mix them all together and boil them a little and put them in a glass vessel well stopped and put thereof three spoonfuls into a potel of good wine and mix it well together.*

*"When it is needed, let him that shall be cut sit against a good fire and make him drink thereof until he fall asleep and then you may safely cut him, and when you have done your cure and will have him awake, take vinegar and salt and wash well his temples and his cheekbones and he shall awake immediately."*[26]

The Jewish historian Flavius Josephus (30-100 A.D.) reports that, the *Baaras*(mankdrake), had only one virtue, that of expelling demons from sick persons, as the demons cannot bear either its smell or its presence (Wars of the Jews, book vii, cap. vi.).

One of the more distasteful subjects is the lore of the Mandrake, that is to be collected from the beneath the hanging gallows. It was believed that the issue of the criminal would produce the finest quality plant for all things magical.

The occultist rock-band *Deep Purple* sings praise of its ability to cause lust in a song called *Mandrake Root* on their 1968 album *Shades of Deep Purple*.

> "I've got a Mandrake Root
> It's some thunder in my brain
> I feed it to my babe
> She thunders just the same
> ***Food of love sets her flame***
> Ah, stick it up

---

[26] *Dwale Manuscript*. Syndics of Cambridge University Library (MS Dd.6.29, f79r-v) cited in: Dwale: an anaesthetic from old England: Anthony J Carter, Department of Anaesthetics, North Staffordshire Hospital, Stoke on Trent ST4 6QG BMJ. 1999 December 18; 319(7225): 1623-1626. Copyright © 1999, British Medical Journal

I've got the Mandrake Root
Baby's just the same
She still feels a quiver
She's still got the flame
She slows down, slows right down
I've got the power"


John Donne(1572-1631) an English poet

*Go and catch a falling star,*
*Get with child a mandrake root,*
*Tell me where all past years are,*
*Or who cleft the devils foot;*


THE TALES AND NOVELS
OF
J. DE LA FONTAINE

Volume 15.

*The remedy all obstacles removed;*
   *'Tis from the root of certain tree expressed;*
   *A juice most potent ev'ry where confessed,*
   *And Mandrake called, which taken by a wife;*
   *More pow'r evinces o'er organick life,*
   *Than from conventual grace was e'er derived,*
   *Though in the cloister youthful friars hived.*

   *TEN months from hence I'll you a father make;*
   *No longer time than that I ask to take;*
   *This period o'er, the child to church we'll bring,-*
   *If true, said Nicia, what a glorious thing!*

### Henbane

Henbane was the secret ingredient in the much desired "love potion" of fame. It inflamed one's passions of the flesh, and made the mind weak and easily bent to another's will. In the days when virginity was priceless, once a maid was "had", marriage was a sure bet to keep things quiet.[27]

Henbane was also the flying herb of witches. After blending the herb with ingredients from bat's blood, to vipers, or toads, and the fat of dead children[28], the witch would rub the mixture into her skin. Soon the witch would start to hallucinate, imagining that she was soaring through the air or dancing with demons. Some believe this enabled them to pierce "the veil" of the spirit world and interact with the demons of the netherworld.

Henbane is mentioned most famously in Sir Richard Burton's *The Arabian Nights*:

*"Presently he filled a cresset with firewood, on which he strewed powdered henbane, and lighting it, went round about the tent with it till the smoke entered the nostrils of the guards, and they all fell asleep, drowned by the drug."*

## Nightshades at War

In 200 B.C., Carthaginian defenders of the city withdrew, leaving behind large quantities of wine that was laced with mandrakes. When the invading Romans drank the wine, they became insensible. Then the Carthaginians returned to destroy them.[29]

---

[27] *The Witch's Herb Garden*
[28] *Witchcraft in England*, Christina Hole
[29] *The Silent Weapon - Poisons and Antidotes in the Middle Ages* by Gunnora Hallakarva.

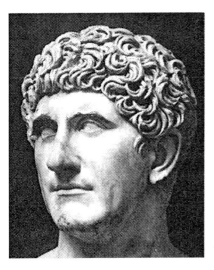

*Marc Anthony* (83-30 b.c.)

Atropine was even used to poison the troops of Marc Anthony in the Parthian Wars. Modern medicine is now able to return to historical writings and identify the plants used by the behaviors exhibited by those poisoned.

*The Datura stramonium (Mandrake) referred to by Dr. Lai has poisonous seeds and berries, with hyoscine a major constituent. Although in toxic doses it almost always ensured insensibility before death, if an extract was given in smaller amounts it had a sedative and possibly aphrodisiac effect. Toxic effects of Datura may have been responsible for the losses suffered by Mark Anthony's army in 36 C.E., when his troops were forced to eat unfamiliar plants, and they "ate of one plant that killed them after driving them mad."[30]*

The same was added to the wine that Macbeth gave the Danes during a "truce."[31] It has been a dreaded poison for quite a long time.

As long as we are talking about Marc Anthony: When Cleopatra wanted to leave this world for the next, she tested various poisons, by using slaves and prisoners. Strychnine effectiveness was disregarded because it twisted the facial features. No one likes an ugly corpse.

Next, she tested deadly nightshade; the first thing noticed was the dilation of the pupils. However lovely her eyes might be from the nightshade berries, the rapid and painful death was too much for the queen. She decided that spending her last moments experiencing rapid respiration, disorientation, and convulsions to be undesirable. In the end she hired a cobra to do the deed; 15 minutes later, she stopped breathing.[32]

---

[30] *Anesthetic Uses of Hyoscine and Atropine Alkaloids in Surgical Arabic Book*; Holzman, Robert S. MD; Anesthesiology:Volume 90(6)June 1999pp 1795-1796
31 *Solanine*, Davey Stoker, Lincoln College, Oxford University.
32. *"Good Witch Hunting."*, Schwarcz, Joe, Canadian Chemical News, July 1, 2001.COPYRIGHT 2001 Chemical Institute of Canada

*"Give me to drink mandragora (mandrake)...*
*That I might sleep out this great gap of time*
*My Antony is away."*
-Shakespeare: Antony and Cleopatra, i. 5.

Now we return to warfare:

Duncan, the 84th King of Scotland (AD 1034-1040), used wine dosed with "sleepy nightshade" against the troops of Sweno, King of Norway. When the battle had ceased near Culross, King Duncan started negotiations for surrender, sending messengers to Sweno. The Scots brought with them "gifts" for the Norwegians to ease the discussions. Of course the Norwegians thought victory was at hand, as the Scots were asking for mercy. The Norwegians they lowered their guard and drank the "laced" wine, which rendered them ineffective for battle. Thus the Scottish forces under the command of Bancho crushed the invaders.[33,34]

In 1672 the Bishop of Muenster, Bernhard van Galen, assaulted the city of Groningen for six weeks. It was successfully defended by Carel Rabenhaupt in heroic style. The *"Bombing Berend"* used projectiles armed with Deadly Nightshade to sicken the defenders. The missiles would catch fire and produce a black and toxic smoke. Apparently, the Bishop's prayers were unheard: the wind changed direction, driving the smoke upon his own troops, bringing their own retreat. It was this battle that led to a treaty between the French and Germans, outlawing such chemical weapons in warfare.[35] Called the Strasbourg Agreement, it included an article banning

---

33 Buchanan G; Watkins J, trans. *The History of Scotland.* London, England: HenryFisher, Son, and P. Jackson; 1831. Cited in: Goodman E. The Descriptive Toxiclogy ofAtropine. Edgewood Arsenal, Md. Unpublished manuscript, 1961.

34 Lewin L. Die Gifte in der Weltgeschichte. Berlin, Germany: Julius Springer; 1920: 537-538. Cited in: Goodman E. The Descriptive Toxicology of Atropine. Edgewood Arsenal,Md. Unpublished manuscript, 1961.

35 Lewin L. Die Gifte in der Weltgeschichte. Berlin, Germany: Julius Springer; 1920: 537-563. Cited in: Goodman E. *The Descriptive Toxicology of Atropine.* Edgewood Arsenal,Md. Unpublished manuscript, 1961.

the use of "perfidious and odious" toxic devices. They would both ignore this treaty later in World War I.

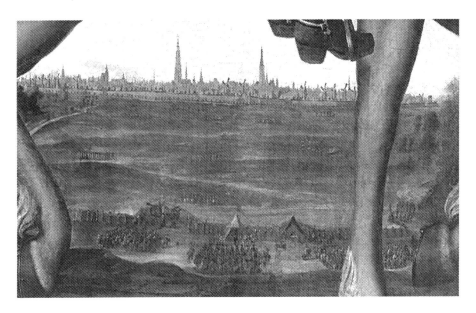

**The Battle of Groningen**

In one of the oddest of stories of nightshades in warfare is the case of the French soldiers in 1813 who had invaded the starving locals, (*the location is not mentioned but is most likely Napoleon's troops during the retreat of the Battle of Vitoria, June 21, 1813*). The soldiers found themselves starving along with the local peasants, and ate Deadly Nightshade berries. The company surgeon, Gaultier, recorded the events, (general confusion, self-destruction by wandering around half-naked in swamps, and throwing themselves into campfires.)[36] Now, this is considered positive behavior by certain libertine groups.

In February of 1881, Lieutenant-Colonel Flatters was marching his French troops from Algeria to the Sudan, by way of the Tuareg people's territory. These are called "the Blue Men" or "the People of Veil", who in

---

36 *INCAPACITATING AGENTS*, JAMES S. KETCHUM, M.D., ABPN*; AND FREDERICK R. SIDELL, M.D.

contrast to other Muslims, veiled men rather than women. Others called these men "the Abandoned of God."

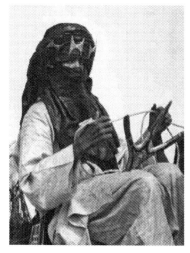

*Image: modern Tuareg*

Flatters, against a warning from the Tuareg, continued to march. He was ambushed on February 16, losing approximately 60 of 120 men. Afterwards the Tuareg, two hundred strong, followed him as he continued to march to a French Outpost.

By the 8th of March, supplies low, they met with three men who said they were not Tuareg. From these men they bought "dried dates." After the troops consumed them, they quickly showed signs of nightshade poisoning. Of the 36 men, five disappeared within five minutes, the rest were so ill that they were incapacitated. Some crawled into the desert, others were tied down by those who had not eaten the "dates". In the morning they were somewhat recovered, "...they set off, half mad, bent double under excruciating pain, their legs crumbling away under them, their voices shrill, their words unintelligible." Chemical warfare at its best: have your enemy pay for their own destruction.

On day two, they came upon an oasis, where the Tuareg were waiting in ambush. Most illness had worn off and they were able to fight, and defended themselves after a bitter battle the Tuareg retreated. They were able to find water and survived by way of cannibalism. Only 12 now remained to finally report to the French Outpost.

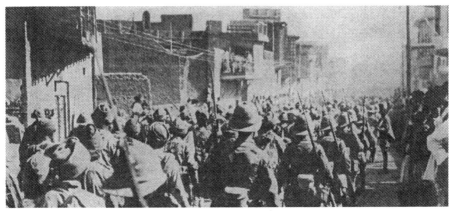

*French troops marching Turkish prisoners down*
*New Street, Bagdad, Iraq, W.W I*
*Photo: www.worldwarone.com*

The French soldiers would again be attacked with nightshades in Vietnam. On the 27 of June, 1908, in Hanoi, North Vietnam, two hundred French soldiers were poisoned by datrua, in their evening meal. The soldiers reported various hallucinations, one saw ants in his bed, another climbed a tree to escape a tiger, one shot at birds in the sky, none of which existed. Two native troops were convicted of plotting with ex-river pirates who were working with the "Chinese reformers/agitators."[37,38]

---

[37] The Times. London, England: 3 July 1908:8; 9 July 1908:7. Cited in: Goodman E. *The Descriptive Toxicology of Atropine.* Edgewood Arsenal, Md. Unpublished manuscript,1961.
[38] Lewin L. Gifte und Vergiftungen. Berlin, Germany: Georg Stilke; 1929: 809. Cited in:Goodman E. *The Descriptive Toxicology of Atropine.* Edgewood Arsenal, Md. Unpublished manuscript, 1961.

## Medical Use

This compound, however, has the ability to be used for good or evil. Atropine is considered a clean drug, meaning without malicious side effects, and is used in many necessary medicines. Dioscorides, an ancient Greek physician, pharmacologist and botanist who practiced in Rome at the time of Nero, circa 40 A.D., alludes to the employment of mandrakes to produce anesthesia when patients are cut or burnt.

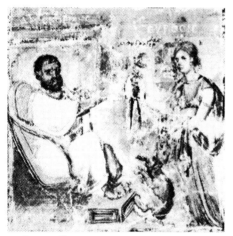

*Dioscorides receiving mandrake from the nymph Epinoia*[39]

Pliny the Elder, a Roman statesman, circa 23 A.D., refers to the odor of mandrakes as causing sleep if it was taken *"before cuttings and puncturings lest they be felt"*. Lucian speaks of mandrakes used before the application of the cautery. Galen of Pergamum, an ancient Greek physician (AD 129 – 200), has a short allusion to its power to paralyze sense and motion. Isidorus (Cartagena, Spain, about 560 – April 4, 636), is quoted as saying: "A wine of the bark of the root is given to those about to undergo operation, that being asleep they may feel no pain."

Ugone da Lucca, who was born in the middle of the twelfth century, discovered a soporific (sleeping agent) which, on being inhaled, put patients to sleep so that they were insensible to pain during operations—the agent he employed was mandrakes. [40]

---

[39] From *Juliana Anicia* Codex 1512. Source: Raphael (1979)

[40] 1914 Catholic Encyclopedia

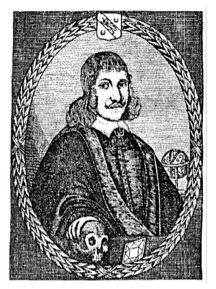

*Nicholas Culpeper*

Culpeper (1616-1654) was an herbalist of his time. He spoke out against England's College of Physicians, calling them self-serving, greed-crazed hypocrites. Same song still heard today, oddly enough. One of his accusations was that they were giving out drugs, without properly testing them.

*"The juice dropped into the ears, eases pains thereof that arise of heat of inflammations. And Pliny saith, it is good for hot swellings under the throat. Have a care you mistake not the deadly Nightshade for this; if you know it not, you may let them both alone, and take no harm, having other medicines sufficient in the book."* – The English Physician by Nicholas Culpeper

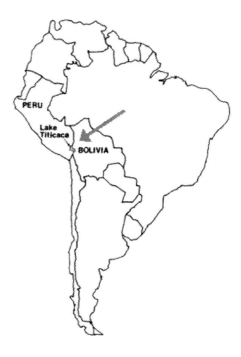

## Potatoes in America–I feel bad

Potatoes themselves were only known to the Incas of Peru and Chile, until the Spanish invaded in the 1600's. Recently, *"Agricultural Research Service botanist David M. Spooner has uncovered DNA evidence showing that early potatoes also came from South America's southwestern coast, in lowland Chile."*[41] Some think Lake Titicaca, Peru is the origin of Potatoes. It is believed that they started to cultivate the potato in 200 B.C. Some historians say that this is the prayer of the Incas for the potato:

*"O Creator! Thou who givest life to all things and hast made men that they may live, and multiply. Multiply also the fruits of the earth, the potatoes and other food that thou hast made, that men may not suffer from hunger and misery."*[42]

---

41 Agricultural Research Service botanist David M. Spooner *"New clues to origin of potatoes."*, M2 Presswire, March 18, 2005.
42 *History of Potato*, 2004 by Linda Stradley

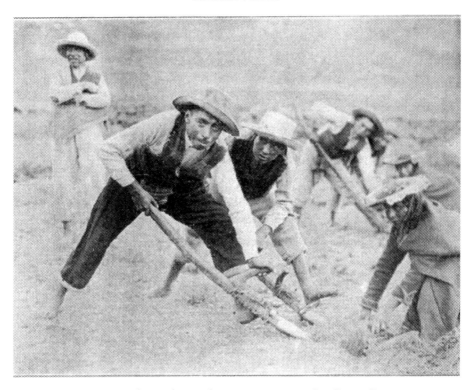

*Inca descendants plowing potatoes in La Raya, Peru*

The Incas would place raw slices on broken bones to quicken healing. They thought if you carried one around it would help with rheumatism. Potatoes were used to make childbirth easier.[43] They even measured time by the how long it took to cook a tater. It's tater time! Instead of minutes I guess they had "taters". Maybe you would see the sign on the local witchdoctor's door, "back in five taters," or hear him exclaim, "I'll be with you in just a tater."

In 1540, Spaniards encountered the people of Central America. It was during this time that the Old World discovered the potato. The Spanish brought it over from Peru to Seville, most likely by the sailors, and

---

[43] History Magazine - *The Impact of the Potato*, Jeff Chapman

not the government. For about 200 years most of Western Europe would not touch it.[44]

## The Royal Treatment

In the following history, you will see how the governors of counties tricked or forced potatoes on to the people. The people rejected them and would at times rebel. Potatoes are now considered a normal food, but only 300 years ago this was not the case. At first, they collected these plants as ornamentals and not as a food; if it was food it was only for slaves, and the Incas were slaves in the eyes of Spanish. These early discoverers of the potato noted that the Incas would take the potatoes to the highest points of the hilltops, place them upon rocks and crush them with their feet and allow them to dry in the sun for long periods of time. This practice would have greatly increased the toxins in the potatoes, as solanine content increases when potatoes are exposed to light. According to William McNeill, the earliest known record showing that potatoes were being grown in Europe dates from 1588 when Carolus Clusius made a watercolor of what he called "Papas Peruanorum."[45]

*Sir Walther Raleigh*

The first Europeans to eat what the Spanish called "the edible stone" were the unfortunate Irish. It was the sworn and bloody enemy of the Irish, Sir Walter Raleigh (1552-1618), who thrust this plague upon these poor people in 1589. He took part in the suppres-

---

[44] Larry Zuckerman, *The Potato-How the humble little spud rescued the western world.*, Interview, KUOW Seattle, 8/24/1998; Publication: Morning Edition (NPR); Author: Renee Montagne, Washington, DC

[45] William McNeill is Professor Emeritus in the Department of History, University of Chicago. Plagues and Peoples (1976) and The Global Tradition: Conquerors, Catastrophes and Community (1992).

sion of the Desmond Rebellions. He was present at the Siege of Smerwick, Ireland, where he oversaw the slaughter of some 600-700 Italian soldiers, which has been sent by the Vatican to protect the Irish Catholics from the English Protestants. The majority were beheaded in a nearby field over two days, including women and children, after they had surrendered unconditionally.[46]

The introduction of potatoes did not happen without some troubles; legend has it that Raleigh made a gift of the potato plant to Queen Elizabeth I (1533-1603).[47] The gentry were invited to a grand banquet featuring potatoes in every course. The cooks, never having seen potatoes before, tossed out the tubers and then boiled stems and leaves (highly poisonous), which promptly made everyone deathly ill. The potatoes were banned from court,[48] and immediately given to the Irish.

Queen Elizabeth I gave Raleigh 40,000 acres of land near Cork, Ireland, in order to raise potatoes for the recently oppressed Irish. A most interesting activity for someone who banned them after being poisoned by them. Accused of treason by Elizabeth's successor, James I, who distrusted him, Raleigh was imprisoned in the Tower of London and eventually put to death.[49]

He is better know for the introduction of tobacco, the famous Raleigh Cigarettes, and Raleigh, North Carolina of tobacco fame are named after him. As mentioned before, tobacco is a nightshade like as potatoes and the rest, in fact they all contain solanine and they all contain nicotine. Yes, the little pile of mashed taters on your plate contains the known carcinogen nicotine, but in far less amounts.

---

[46] Oxford Dictionary of National Biography, online ed., Oxford University Press, Oct 2006,

[47] William H. McNeill disputes this, citing it was a Spanish seaman and not Raleigh. His work: The Introduction of the Potato into Ireland, The Journal of Modern History, Vol. 21, No. 3 (Sep., 1949), pp. 218-222

[48] History of Potato, 2004 by Linda Stradley

[49] "Raleigh, Sir Walter." Encyclopædia Britannica. 2007. Encyclopædia Britannica Online. 24 Jan. 2007 <http://www.britannica.com/eb/article-9062546>.

One of the factors in the introduction of tobacco was the man who it is named after. Jean Nicot (pronounced niko hence nicotine) was born in France, about 1530, in the city of Paris. Employed as the keeper of the Great Seal of France, he later became the private secretary to the King of France, and ambassador to Portugal.

He was a friend of the scholar and botanist Damião de Goes, who showed Nicot the wondrous healing power of tobacco. Goes claimed it was able to cure cancer by direct application to tumors. Nicot tried it out on the face of one his friends for 10 days and voila! The tumors went away. By 1560, Nicot had convinced the King and others of the wonders of tobacco. It became famous when snuff was given to the Queen of France, Catherine de Medici, in order to treat her migraine headaches. It then became the Queen's Herb.[50]

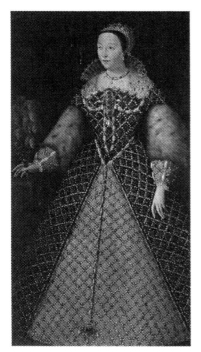

*Catherine de Medici*

What was to happen has been infamous throughout history. Once this cheap food was introduced to the peasant Irish, it enabled the English to reduce the wages of the working class to such paltry amounts that the only food they could afford was the potato. These could be easily grown at home by the feeblest of folks.

---

[50] *A BRIEF CHRONOLOGY OF TOBACCO IN THE CIVILIZED WORLD* by Thomas E. Addison, MD

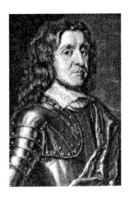

*Cromwell*

The expansion of potato cultivation rested entirely with landless laborers, renting tiny plots from "new" landowners, many of whom were now English, whose interests rested in cattle. It was England's plan to displace the Catholic Irish with Protestants by giving the land confiscated from the oppressed Irish[51] to the veterans of the Cromwellian wars (1649-52). Many of the Irish were landless "tinkers"[52] because of this illegal confiscation of land by the English; my own Great-Grandfather admits to this in his early accounts of those times, his family being one of the new landowners in Ireland.[53]

Now being Irish myself, from "me dear mother", and victim of the wrath of the potato, it seems right to alert the Irish to this trickery of potatoes. In America, we would be tossing them off ships, as *"quick as tea,"* had we known then.

The introduction of potatoes created a sort of economic slavery or bait and switch for the people of Ireland. They thought they were getting cheap food, but in reality their wages would be lowered. This in turn would lower the cost of the food raised by the Irish laborers and sold to the English. It was the English that ended up with the cheap food, a true Trojan Horse if there ever was one.

---

[51] *How the Potato Changed the World's History*, 3/22/1999; Social Research; MCNEILL, WILLIAM H.

[52] Tinkers were non-land owning Irish who would earn a living by fixing pots, pans and other such work.

[53] *Life's Adventure*, by John Brereton, Out of print

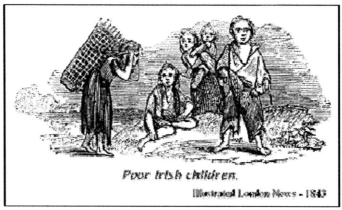

*Before the Famine*

### Thomas Ruggles, *Annals of Agriculture,* 1792

*However, failure to implement this level of wages may, perhaps, be mitigated by the adoption by the poor of the potato, a nutritious and cheap substitute. Nonetheless, the poor will not eat potatoes if they can get anything else, for the daintiness and ignorance of the poor in regard to the wonderments of this root has been the chief obstacle to its adoption.*

### Ralph Leycester, *Annals of Agriculture,* Vol. 29, 1798

*It is with great satisfaction that I can report that wages are now 8s. per week, having only increased 1s. in twenty-five years, and that, considering the use of potatoes and turnips, the laborer is better off than before. Potatoes are in great use here, which necessarily lessens the consumption of bread.*

### *Report of the Devon Commission for Ireland,* 1845

*The potato enabled a large family to live on food produced in great quantities at a trifling cost, and, as the result, the increase of the people has been gigantic.*

Then a tragedy happened, which I cannot imagine saddened the heart of the English at that time. That was the Great Potato Blight of 1845. More than a million Irish, or about 10% of the total population died. A famine of this magnitude was unprecedented and unimaginable in the preceding 200 years. [54]

The Irish had become more and more dependent on the potato as food. So much so, that potatoes were eaten at all three meals per day. Potatoes were considered a wonder food that prevented scurvy and provided good nutrition. They were easy to grow, required almost no training in farming, and used extremely simple technology: just a spade (shovel) was needed. Potatoes stored remarkably well, in cellars that could be easily dug. Cultivation of potatoes could be done by mere children, required no ox or plow, no threshing equipment, or even the purchase of good seed.

*Irish Potato Farmer*

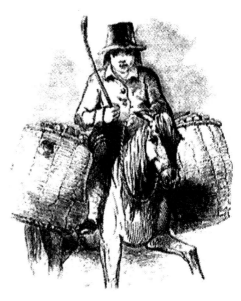

Potatoes also produced more calories per acre than any other food that could be grown. This was a real boon to the poor of Ireland, as one acre of potatoes could easily sustain an entire family. The Irish population doubled to eight million between 1780 and 1841 with no other influence in industry or agricultural intervention other than the cultivation of potatoes. [55]

Just before the great potato famine hit, historians estimate that approximately 30% or 3 million of the inhabitants of Ireland were living nearly exclusively on potatoes as the staple food. The potato of choice at that time, known as the Lumper, had the highest growth and largest size of the other potatoes; it

---

[54] William McNeill is Professor Emeritus in the Department of History, University of Chicago. His works include Plagues and Peoples (1976) and The Global Tradition: Conquerors, Catastrophes and Community (1992).
[55] History Magazine - *The Impact of the Potato*, Jeff Chapman

was also the worst tasting. Many had warned that relying on a single crop might be asking for trouble, but the state of poverty demanded reliance on potatoes. Formerly, the poor who owned land had grown wheat, rye, and other vegetable crops.

When the first blight hit the some of the crop escaped–so most were able to make it through the winter. In the spring, potatoes that were still good were replanted for the new crop. When it rained the blight reappeared; the effects were devastating–this time the entire crop failed. The Great Irish Famine followed. Many died, many left, all suffered.

The cause of this blight was a fungus called *Phytophthora infestans* that had been accidentally imported from North America. [56] Most of the potato crops rotted in the fields, and because potatoes could not be stored longer than 12 months, there was no surplus to fall back on.

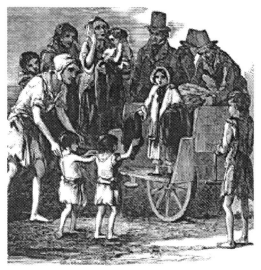

*Giving aid during the Famine*

To give an idea of how much the Irish depended on the potatoes before the blight: the average person was eating between seven and 14 pounds per day. According to a book by Cecil Woodham-Smith on the subject: *"...cooking any food other than a potato had become a lost art. Women*

---

[56] *The Irish Potato Famine*, by Catharina Japikse, [EPA Journal - Fall 1994]

*hardly boiled anything but potatoes. The oven had become unknown after the introduction of the potato prior to the Great Starvation."[57]*

Over 2 million acres of potatoes had been planted in 1845 and within two years the crops were down to 300,000 acres. [58]

What is not noted in history is that all the other crops that were raised in Ireland were not affected[59] by the potato blight. The corn, wheat, barley, rye, and common vegetables continued to grow in the fertile plains. However, this food was no longer affordable for the peasant and was shipped off to England, while the Irish starved. They no longer controlled their own country, or their own fate. This caused the great Irish migration, as the peasants looked for better lands to live in, such as America–where they would face the NINA movement.

*The New York Times, March 25, 1854*

W. COLE, No. 8 Ann-st.

GROCERY CART AND HARNESS FOR SA
—In good order, and one chestnut horse, 8 years old
excellent saddle horse; can be ridden by a lady. Also,
young man wanted, from 16 to 18 years of age, able to w
No Irish need apply. CLUFF & TUNIS, No. 270 W
ington-st., corner of Myrtle-av., Brooklyn.

BILLIARD TABLE FOR SALE—Of Leom
manufacture; been used about nine months. Also,
tures of a Bar-room. Inquire on the premises. No.

---

[57] *The Great Hunger: Ireland 1845-1849* by Cecil Woodham-Smith
[58] *The Irish Potato Famine,* by Catharina Japikse, [EPA Journal - Fall 1994]
[59] N.I.N.A. No Irish Need Apply. This was the attitude the Irish immigrants would face when looking for work in America.

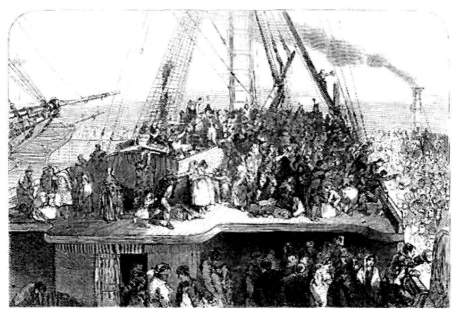

THE DEPARTURE.

*The Departure: Leaving Ireland Forever*

The potato went to Italy and England about 1585, to Belgium and Germany by 1587, to Austria about 1588, and to France around 1600. Wherever the potato was introduced, it was considered foul, poisonous, and downright evil. How wise were those peasants.

The potato was thought to cause all sorts of diseases including leprosy, but also syphilis, narcosis, scrofula, early death, sterility, and rampant sexuality, and to destroy the soil where it grew. The spud was so hated that in the town of Besancon, France a law was passed stating: *"In view of the fact that the potato is a pernicious substance whose use can cause leprosy, it is hereby forbidden, under pain of fine, to cultivate it."* [60] It should be noted that earlier I mentioned Henbane and Shakespeare, where he made a connection with leprosy and Henbane. It might be wise to not consider them foolish in this regard, as the term; leprosy may have had a wider meaning than it has today. Many words have changed meaning remarkably even in one generation, such as "cool" or "hot" a reference to style, rather than heat. That

---

[60] *History of Potato*, 2004 by Linda Stradley

being said, neither nightshades nor Henbane cause leprosy as we know it today.

Antoine Augustine Parmentier ( 1737-1813 ), a French agricultural engineer in the French military of the 18th century, was captured by the Prussians.[61] He tasted the potato in a prisoner of war camp, during the Seven Years' War (1756-1763) and instantly recognized its properties as a staple. The other prisoners, however, refused to eat potatoes; they had to be cooked down into a soup so the prisoners did not know what they were eating.

After returning home Parmentier planted potatoes in France, but people considered them to be unhealthy and would not eat them. He then went to see the King and convinced him of their properties with his study of the potato called *Chemical Examination of the Potato*.[62] King Louis XVI, realizing he needed to provide food for the starving masses, planted a field of potatoes and started publishing recipes in newspapers, having Potato Parties, even Potato Fashion, but the people would not fall for it. They refused to eat them, as they knew potatoes were related to the Deadly Nightshade Plant, having the same flowers.

So the King tricked them. He put guards around a field of potatoes, so no one could steal the King's tubers. This wise king also doubled the guard during the day, but would relax it during the night. This aroused curiosity among the people and they wanted to taste this new food; if it is worth guarding it is worth stealing. They stole them during the night, and proceeded to dine upon the King's tubers. That was how he convinced the population to eat potatoes. Interestingly, Ben Franklin dined at Parmentier's home and was treated to course after course of potato-based dishes, up to and including a potato-based after-dinner liqueur.[63]

---

[61] 1914 Catholic Encyclopedia

[62] *History of Potato*, 2004 by Linda Stradley

[63] History Magazine - *The Impact of the Potato*, Jeff Chapman

"Let them eat cake!"[64] Those were the words of the Royalty, as potatoes were smashed into little cakes at the time. Whether it was England, Germany or France; the new peasant food had arrived.

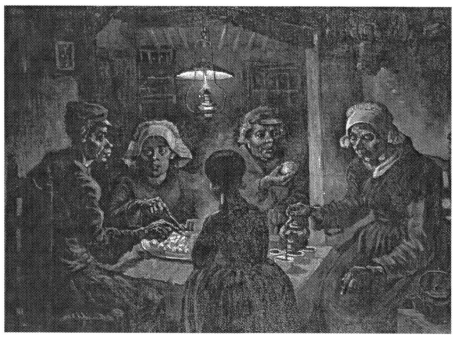

*The Potato Eaters* (Van Gogh Museum, Amsterdam; 1885)

This painting depicted a social class that could be distinguished by the food that it ate. As potatoes took favor, the poor relied on it more and more as a staple.

In Corsica, General Pascal Paoli, the great reformer, introduced them to the people there. His enemies then gave him the title "general potato," or General Delle Patate. This, however, was not a compliment, as most of the world still considered the potato poisonous.

---

[64] Many argue over the exact meaning of this phrase; some think it was the crust of ovens that was called cake while others say it was potato cakes. The saying is attributed to Marie Antoinette, who also wore potato flowers in her hair at the time.

The same pressure was applied by King Frederick William I (1712 to 1786) of Germany. He first issued an order in 1774 for his subjects to grow potatoes as protection against famine. The town of Kolberg replied: *'The things have neither smell nor taste, not even the dogs will eat them, so what use are they to us?'* The King issued an edict to the people who refused to plant and cultivate the potato, that transgressors would suffer the removal of their noses and ears.[65]

In the early 1800s the Socialists and the first Governor of Greece, Ioannis Kapodistrias, introduced potatoes to the populace. The people of Greece were not impressed by this new food. The government put out great tables of potatoes, for nearly free, in the public squares, but these were refused by the people. Then taking the invidious strategy of the French they raised the price, and placed guards around them. This caused the people to think that they were extremely rare and valuable, so they began to steal them and grow them at home.

In 1805 potatoes were introduced by the French to Serbia. Earlier potatoes had been introduced along with tobacco to the United States by our old friend Sir Walter Raleigh. So when you see people dying from emphysema you can thank Sir Walter Raleigh for making tobacco popular. Other sources say the first potatoes were brought to America in 1621 at Jamestown, Virginia, when the Governor of Bermuda, Nathaniel Butler, sent them to the Governor of Jamestown, Francis Wyatt.[66] Russian fur traders also brought them to Alaska from Siberia in 1783. By 1890, potatoes became an industry in Maine.

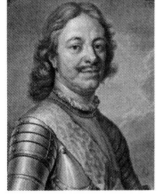

*Peter the Great*

Potatoes were introduced in Russia by Peter the Great. Czarina Catherine gave orders to mandate the cultivation of potatoes. This

---

[65] According to History Magazine - *The Impact of the Potato*, Jeff Chapman, the King of Prussia used the same trick as the King of France in order to introduce them.
[66] History Magazine - The Impact of the Potato, Jeff Chapman

was quickly stopped, momentarily, by the Russian Orthodox, who rightly considered them a poisonous food not suitable for consumption by the people. They called them "Devil's apples" or the fruit of witches. In 1840, the government issued another decree ordering peasants to plant potatoes on common lands. This resulted in a series of "potato riots," which led the government to stop forcing cultivation of the potato, but the little spud had started to grow on the hungry peasants–because of famine.[67]

As potatoes were introduced to the peoples of Europe, the peasant class refused to eat them, as they understood families of plants by their flowers and leaves. Knowing that *atropine belladonna* was a poisonous plant and that potatoes had the same flower, they rightly connected the dots. Finally, in 1850 Czar Nicholas I enforced Czarina Catherine's orders with his troops and the rest is history. [68]

Some of the more compelling reasons for the introduction of potatoes to the peasant population were famine and wars. Many of the European countries were barely able to grow enough grains to support themselves throughout the year. If rains came to spoil the rye or wheat, the entire year was lost and famine would ensue. The ability's of potatoes to grow in poor seasons and be stored for nearly a year made it a wonder crop. Potatoes could yield nearly 2 to 4 times the amount of calories per acre, than the grain crops.

The Napoleonic wars often had troops fighting in fields and destroying crops. With grain crops, there is only a short season for planting and once the crop is destroyed, the year is a bust. Whereas the potato plants could be trampled under the feet of soldiers and the tubers would remain intact. The tops of the potato plant are far more resilient than are any of the grains to such treatment.

Moisture can cause an infection (ergot) to grow on rye which creates the drug-like effect of LSD, which could send entire villages into temporary mania. Rodents would often raid the grain storage bins, and so would hungry soldiers. Potatoes, however, could be hidden underground; the rodents refused to touch them and the soldiers refused to dig for them. All of this led to the future popularity of potatoes.

---

[67] Utenkova, Yelena. *Potatoes in uniform*, Russian Life, November 1, 1997.
[68] History Magazine - *The Impact of the Potato*, Jeff Chapman

On the contrary, in warmer climates potatoes would store poorly as soon as the warm weather hit; little sprouts would grow whether they were in the ground or in storage bins. In warmer weather, potatoes would also rot. When grain is stored tightly in jars, it can be stored for many a year. This is one of the reasons the potatoes were more popular in the cooler northern climates such as Poland, Russia and Ireland. [69]

During the Alaskan Klondike gold rush, (1897-1898) potatoes were literally worth their weight in gold, as the valuable *vitamin C* was greatly needed by the miners. Potatoes were also valuable there for their long storage capabilities. On the island of Tristan de Cunha in South America potatoes were the unofficial currency (the tater traders...).

In 1801-1809 Thomas Jefferson made French Fries popular by serving them at the White House while president. [70]

In the 1850's most Americans considered the potato as food for animals rather than for humans. As late as the middle of the 19th Century, the Farmer's Manual recommended that potatoes "be grown near the hog pens as a convenience towards feeding the hogs." [71]

It is rumored that in 1853 the great railroad tycoon, Commodore Cornelius Vanderbilt, at an upper class resort in Saratoga Springs, NY, sent an order of potatoes back to the cook that had been cut too thickly. Of course, this did not go over well with the Chef. In a fit of revenge, he sliced the potatoes paper-thin and fried them in oil, added a dash of salt, and thus created the first potato chips, known then as "Saratoga Crunch Chips."

Not everyone was pleased with the introduction of potatoes as food. Some even noticed the ill effects they have on cattle.

*"It is generally supposed that the water in which potatoes are boiled is injurious; and as instances are recorded where cattle having drunk it were seriously*

---

[69] *How the Potato Changed the World's History*, 3/22/1999; Social Research; MCNEILL, WILLIAM H.

[70] History Magazine - *The Impact of the Potato*, Jeff Chapman

[71] *History of Potato*, 2004 by Linda Stradley

*affected, it may be well to err on the safe side, and avoid its use for any alimentary (eating) purpose."[72]* Isabella Beeton's 1862 Book of Household Management

*"Nor do I say it is filthy to eat potatoes. I do not ridicule the using of them as a sauce. What I laugh at is, the idea of the use of them being a saving; of their going further than bread; of the cultivating of them in lieu of wheat adding to the human sustenance of a country....As food for cattle, sheep or hogs, this is the worst of all the green and root crops; but of this I have said enough before; and therefore, I now dismiss the Potato with the hope, that I shall never again have to write the word, or see the thing."* -William Cobbett (1763-1835), British journalist and reformer

In the early nineteenth century, potatoes were blamed for making people weak and soft; Ludwig Feuerbach[73] and other German radicals believed that "potato blood" was the reason for the delay of the revolution they wanted in the German people.[74]

---

[72] Ibid

[73] Ludwig Feuerbach, (1804–1872) along with Schopenhauer, Kierkegaard, Marx, and Nietzsche, must be counted among those philosophical outsiders who rebelled against the academic philosophy of the 19th century and thought of themselves as reformers and prophets of a new culture. Although he began his career as an enthusiastic follower of Hegel, he emerged in the 1840's as a leader of the Young Hegelians, a group of radicals who, inspired by the revolutionary political spirit sweeping over Europe, employed the critical side of Hegel's philosophy to undermine the reactionary alliance of philosophy, State, and Christianity in Prussia. But confronted by censorship, the police, and reprisals against them in the universities they turned against Hegel's philosophy altogether. Expelled from the faculties for which they were trained, many of them became pamphleteers, journalists, revolutionaries, and independent scholars. (Van A. Harvey, Stanford Encyclopedia of Philosophy)

[74] *How the Potato Changed the World's History,* 3/22/1999; Social Research; MCNEILL, WILLIAM H.

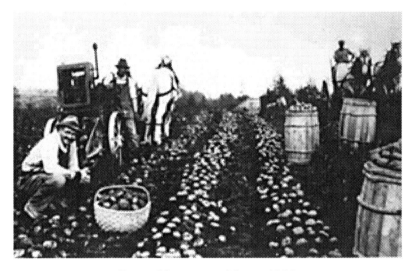

*Potato Harvesting, Maine 1930*

In 1995, the United States sent potatoes into space to see if they would grow there in order to feed future astronauts; it was a joint effort between NASA and the University of Wisconsin, Madison. Space may be the best place for potatoes; the error was in returning them to earth.

Once potatoes were introduced to the people, tomatoes and egg-plant followed quickly.

Currently Atropine is used by the U.S. Government to combat the effects of Nerve Gas; it is used in surgery and in nasal decongestants to reduce fluid production, to dilate pupils, to treat stomach and bladder cramps. Scopolamine is used for motion sickness and as an "anti-spasmodic." Solanine is not used in medicine but as a commercial pesti-cide. All of these chemicals, neurotoxins, are found in all nightshade plants, even the ones we eat.

Potatoes are now one of world's main sources of food; only wheat is greater. Over one billion people eat potatoes, and half of them are in developing countries. Annual amounts eaten per person vary from country to country. In Europe, it is 80kg, North America 60kg, Latin America 21kg, Asia 12kg, and Africa 8kg. Potatoes are the fourth largest food crop by volume in the world, with global production projected to increase 13%

from an average of 250 million tons per annum in 1987 to more than 300 million tons by the year 2000. [75]

Consumption in third world countries is up too: from 9kg/captia in 1961-63 to 14kg/captia in 1995-97 according to FAOSTAT (June 1998). This is small potatoes (pardon the pun) compared to Europe and Americas, which are at 86kg/captia and 63kg/captia respectively, per annum. The little spud is going global quickly.

What about the tomato? You might ask. Well, the history is much the same; it too was brought over from South America[76] by the Spanish; however, it is not a staple food like the potato. Therefore, its history is of less relevance as people were not kept alive solely by tomatoes. What is interesting is that Mediterranean food, namely Italian, has been completely altered by the introduction of the tomato, which was unknown until the 1800's. Before that, people considered them "wolf apples" (*Solanum lycopersicum*, *lyco* means wolf), and not fit for human consumption. Imagine Italy without pasta sauce; I know it is difficult, but before the tomato they only used olive oil and garlic, pesto, and cheese for pasta. Nor were there peppers or eggplant; the peppers were imported along with tomatoes and potatoes,[77] and the eggplant came from China and India.[78] There are no Greek or Latin references to the eggplant before the 1600's. Eggplant was originally called, *Aubergine*, which has Arabic roots, apparently introduced by the Arab invaders (Islamic-Ottomans) into Persia.

---

[75] John Vandenberg, Horticulture & Special Crops Division, Agriculture & AgriFood Canada, March 10, 1999
[76] *Our Vegetable Travelers* by Victor R. Boswell, August, 1949 issue, Volume 96(2) of National Geographic Magazine

[77] Eshbaugh, W.H. 1993. *History and exploitation of a serendipitous new crop discovery.* p. 132-139. In: J. Janick and J.E. Simon (eds.), New crops. Wiley, New York.
[78] Ibid (Vegetable Travelers)

## Terrorism, Taters, and Tobacco

In more recent years, nightshades have even become weapons of terror. The following is a news report from Fox News on how solanine found in potatoes could be used for terrorism. The Incas would boil down potatoes in order to extract solanine, so it could be used on poison arrows for hunting monkeys. Now the FBI is worried about terrorists boiling down potatoes to hunt Americans.

A recent British find in the home of a follower of Osama bin Laden was a manual of how the warrior of Allah could create poisons for hostages and prisoners.

*"ASSASSINATIONS WITH POISON*

*We will limit the discussion to poisons that the holy warrior can prepare and use without endangering his health... Tobacco. There is enough nicotine in three cigarettes to kill a man. If eaten, sixty to seventy milligrams of pure nicotine will kill a person within an hour. Potato sprout. Both rotten and green, contains solanine. XXXXX can be found with XXXXXX. Mix poison with this substance, and when the enemy touches it he will die slowly within fifteen minutes to an hour. Poisoning from eating spoiled food. Since 0.000028 gram will kill a person, this poison is absolutely lethal."*[79]

---

[79] *"KILLING IS EASY!*(terrorism)(Brief Article)", Harper's Magazine, June 1, 2001.

A friend of mine commented that this information should not be included in this book, as it could be dangerous, my reply was, "This is going on in every kitchen in America, except no one knows they are doing it." So I lined out the important parts, just to be safe–You never know.

(3)

### D. POTATO AND CIGARETTE POISON

A transparent liquid, has a sweet taste, dissolve in ████████████, i.e. potatoes
Cigarette poison: tannish yellow oil
Both tolerate high temperature as in cooking

Potato poison: Lethal dose = 60mlg = 6 drops
Cigarette:                      80mlg
Death  1 to 4 hours
Double dose for immediate death

**Preparation:**

We take 2kg of potatoes, remove the roots, and grind them well. We take the flour and cover it with ████████████████ which is "used for massaging". We cover the flour with ████████████████, and then we cover the receptacle with a plastic bag tied firmly. We place the receptacle in a container of water and heat and stir -- the water boils - for an hour and we take the formed substance in the receptacle, filter and press it well. Evaporate it in the sun for an hour or two, where the ████████████ and remains a liquid namely the poison.

NB: if we leave it for 24 hours before filtering it, the poison will be stronger.
Potato poison "*solajene*"[1] is used in food, drink or cooking.
Nicotine ███████████████████████████████████████████
itself)

4172

---
[1] Phonetically spelled

Image: Maxwell Hutchkinson, *The Poisoner's Handbook*

Thursday, September 04, 2003

## Fox News

WASHINGTON — The FBI has warned law enforcement agencies that terrorists may use nicotine (search) and solanine (search) as "mass poisoning agents."

Nicotine can be obtained from tobacco. Solanine can be obtained from potatoes.

"References to nicotine and solanine appear in numerous terrorist training manuals and documents seized in Afghanistan," the FBI said in its weekly bulletin to law enforcement agencies, which was sent out late Wednesday. "The most likely technique for nicotine or solanine poisoning would be food, beverage or water contamination; however, nicotine can also be absorbed through the skin and mouth and the digestive and respiratory tracts."

...Acute nicotine poisoning will cause central nervous system depression, neuromuscular paralysis, lowered blood pressure, slowed heart rate and death. More common symptoms of nicotine poisoning include nausea, vomiting and abdominal pain, the FBI said.

Common symptoms of solanine poisoning occur two to 24 hours after exposure and include a harsh, scratchy sensation in the mouth, dehydration and drowsiness. Severe cases include cramps and fever -- and can result in coma and death, the FBI said.

...The lethal dose of nicotine is about 40 to 60 milligrams. Solanine occurs naturally in "greened" potatoes, produced when the potato is old or exposed to sunlight for long periods of time, the FBI said. A large dosage of solanine is necessary to be fatal, the bureau said.

Fox News' Anna Stolley contributed to this report.


## Use as pesticides

Potatoes high in glycol-alkaloid content are produced commercially for pesticides. Once harvested potatoes are converted to dust which is then spread over plants as a pesticide and fungicide.

"Both -chaconine and -solanine have pesticidal properties, including antifeedant and fungicidal properties (Beckstrom-Sternberg and Duke, 1997). - Chaconine also has nematicidal properties. -Chaconine and -solanine were effective as larval feeding deterrents for spruce budworm (Choristoneura fumiferana) (Bentley et al., 1984)." [80]

## Nerve Gas and Nightshades

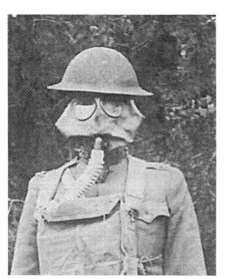

There is a connection between nerve gas and nightshades. The action of the poison of each is the same, but the intensity is quite different. Before we start a little history is fitting about the development of understanding and using cholinesterase inhibitors. World War I saw the first use of modern chemical warfare. The German Army was the first to use chemical weapons; they quietly brought bottles of chlorine gas to the front lines and waited for the right moment when the wind would favor them, then released the gas which drifted across the battlefield toward the French troops. But the wind shifted and returned the gas to the Germans. Even in the face of failure, the use of chemical weapons developed to horrifying dimensions. All of the major powers began to develop and use chemical weapons, especially nerve agents.

Then in 1936, two days before Christmas, Dr. Gerhard Schrader was developing an insecticide for I.G. Farben, when he discovered tabun. As little as 5 parts per million(ppm) killed all of his leaf lice. When he spilled a small drop of tabun, it nearly killed him and his assistant. He

---

[80] a-Chaconine [20562-03-2] and a-Solanine [20562-02-1] Review of Toxicological Literature, Prepared for Errol Zeiger, Ph.D.,National Institute of Environmental Health Sciences,Submitted by Raymond Tice, Ph.D. ,Integrated Laboratory Systems,February 1998

recognized the effects as a nerve disruptor. Soon his new discovery was a Nazi war weapon.

Hitler never used it as he thought the Americans has already discovered it and feared retaliation. However, he was wrong, the Allies did not have any defense against a nerve agent. If Hitler had used tabun, he could, have won the war. I.G. Farben was a major supporter of Nazi movement and worked closely with the Nazis during the invasions so they would gain control of captured chemical plants. They were the developers of the infamous pesticide Zykon-B, an agent used in the Nazi death camp gas chambers at Auschwitz and Majdankek.

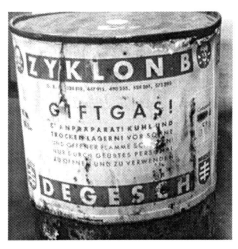

*Photo courtesy of: Stanford University Libraries Academic and Information Resources*

In fact, the death camp at Auschwitz was part of the I.G. Farben chemical plant, where millions were gassed to death.

One of I.G. Farben's conglomerates was Bayer, of aspirin fame; in fact, Dr. Otto Bayer, the research director of I.G. Farben, became a developer of chemical warfare agents for the U.S.

It was discovered that by attacking Acetylcholinesterase(AChE), the nervous system becomes flooded with Acetylcholine(ACh) which causes animals or humans to die quickly. The most famous of this devolved gas is VX Nerve agent, and is considered the world's deadliest chemical[81].

---

[81] The School of Chemistry, University of Bristol

It was the nerve agent used by Saddam Hussein in 1988 when he dropped three VX bombs on Iran, killing 10,000. Dr. Bilal stated that over 157 tons of VX supplies had been destroyed along with 1.5 tons of VX and 10 tons of mustard gas in Iraq.[82] At one time over 800 tons of sarin nerve gas (an irreversible cholinesterase inhibitor) was reported in Iraq.[83]

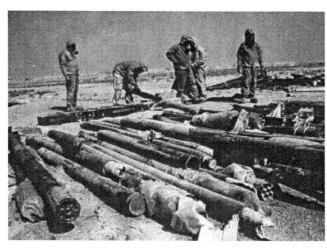

*Nerve gas rockets being prepared for destruction under UN supervision at Khamsiyah, Iraq Photograph courtesy of DSTO*

Nerve agents work by causing sustained contractions of all the muscles in the body, including the diaphragm; the victim dies by asphyxiation. As little as 200 micrograms will kill. The antidote is atropine and pralidoxime. Atropine blocks the receptors of the nerves in the involuntary or smooth muscles, so they will not become severely contracted. This allows breathing until the pralidoxime can regenerate the AChE so the body can begin to function properly.

Solanine found in nightshades is an AChE inhibitor just as is VX; the amounts needed to create the effects are vastly different, but the action is the same. Solanine attacks the AChE the body uses to free ACh from the nerve receptors, as does VX.

---

[82] http://www.globalsecurity.org/wmd/library/report/2004/isg-final-report/isg-final-report_vol3_cw-05.htm
[83] S/1995/284n - UNSCOM Seventh report under resolution 715 10/04/95

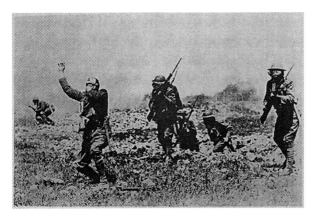

*Phosgene Gas Attack*
*WW I*

The following is an excerpt from a Military Medicine textbook on nerve agents use in chemical warfare. *"Nerve agents inhibit AChE, which then cannot hydrolyze ACh. This classic explanation of nerve agent poisoning holds that the intoxicating effects are due to the excess endogenous Ach."*[84] Solanine has the same effect on the Acetylcholi-nesterase(AChE) in the body as military nerve agents or commercial pesticides, but thankfully not nearly as strong. This will document the fact of the effects of solanine as Acetylcholi-nesterase(AChE) inhibitor and what that exactly means. It is also of note that atropine is found in nightshades and is an agent for treatment for Acetylcholinesterase inhibitors.

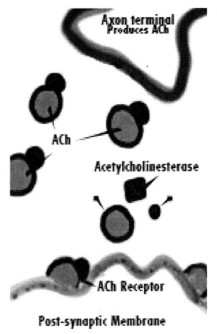

*Figure 1: Normal Activity*

---

[84] Textbook of Military Medicine: *Medical Aspects of Chemical and Biological Warfare*: Chapter 5 ,Nerve Agents, Frederick R. Sidell, M.D.

Once Acetylcholinesterase (AChE) is inhibited this allows the Acetylcholine(ACh) (neurotransmitter) to overstimulate the nervous system. Atropine is used not to combat the nerve agent but to protect the nervous system.

In the following diagrams, you will be able to see the processes involved in the nervous system and the effects of nerve agents like solanine or VX.

*Figure 1* shows the normal activity of the nervous system. Neurotransmitters are released from the Axon terminal and received at the receptor sites. The neurotransmitter is then released by the Acetylcholinesterase so the receptor sites can receive neurotransmitters again. It does this by breaking down the ACh into is separate parts, acetyl and choline. It is then reabsorbed and reused for more neurotransmission.

When a nerve agent (Acetylcholinesterase inhibitor) is introduced, it prevents the Acetylcholinesterase from releasing the neurotransmitters from the receptor sites. When this happens, the body slowly floods with neurotransmitters that must find another place to go, rather than the intended site. This will induce poisoning, by disrupting the function of the nervous system with excess Acetylcholine. This can be seen in Figure 2, where the nerve agent has attacked the Acetylcholinesterase prevents it from functioning, and allows ACh to flood the system.

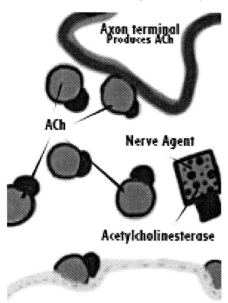

Figure 2: Nerve Agent

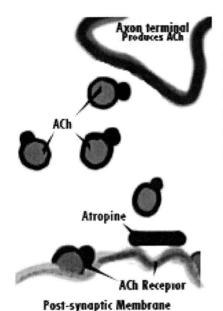

To prevent the receptor sites from activating due to the flooding of neurotransmitters, atropine is administered to nerve agent victims (see figure 3). Atropine attaches to the receptor sites just as neurotransmitters do, but prevents the stimulation of nerves.

*Figure 3: Atropine Blocking Receptors*

**Atropine poisoning:**  Jimson Weed, *Datura* or *loco weed* is a night-shade plant that contains vast quantities of atropine and solanine, and is very deadly.  There is a mnemonic for the physiological effects of atropine intoxication:

*"blind as a bat, mad as a hatter, red as a beet, hot as hell, dry as a bone,*
*the bowel and bladder lose their tone,*
*and the heart runs alone."*

The actual effects are reported to be: cycloplegia (paralysis of the eye muscles) and mydriasis (extreme dilation of the pupil), flushed, warm and dry skin, dry mouth, urinary retention and ileus (slowing or stopping of intestinal movement), rapid heart beat, hypertension or hypotension, and choreoathetosis/jerky movements.  In case of overdose, the effects are hyperthermia, coma, respiratory arrest, and seizures. The vast majority of atropine-poisoning cases are accompanied by delirium with visual and auditory hallucinations.

Tropane alkaloids are some of the few substances which cause "true hallucinations" which cannot be distinguished from reality. This is different from all other hallucinations in which people have distorted vision, or other senses, or understand that they are hallucinating. It may be described as a "real" trance when a user under that influence can be awake but completely disconnected from his immediate environment. In this case, the user would ignore most stimuli and respond to unreal ones. This is unlike psilocybin or LSD, which only cause sensory distortions. The effects of Jimson Weed (*Datura*) have been described as a living dream: consciousness falls in and out, people who don't exist or are miles away are conversed with, etc. The effects can last for days.

The name Jimson Weed (*Datura*) came from Jamestown, Virginia where it was used to poison British soldiers in Bacon's Rebellion. Apparently, the settlers had found out about Jimson Weed's poisonous effects by trying to boil the poison out of the leaves to so they could eat it. However, the plan failed, and they became very sick. This was a desperate measure taken during a time of famine.

*Some of the soldiers sent thither to quell the rebellion of Bacon (1676); and some of them ate plentifully of it, the effect of which was a very pleasant comedy, for they turned natural fools upon it for several days: one would blow up a feather in the air; another would dart straws at it with much fury; and another, stark naked, was sitting up in a corner like a monkey, grinning and making mows [grimaces] at them; a fourth would fondly kiss and paw his companions, and sneer in their faces with a countenance more antic than any in a Dutch droll.*

*In this frantic condition they were confined, lest they should, in their folly, destroy themselves- though it was observed that all their actions were full of innocence and good nature. Indeed, they were not very cleanly; for they would have wallowed in their own excrements, if they had not been prevented. A thousand such simple tricks they played, and after 11 days returned themselves again, not remembering anything that had passed*

*–Robert Beverly, The History and Present State of Virginia, 1705*

*"Satan has ever sought to engraft the deadly nightshade of error upon the life-giving Rose of Sharon"* - THE INNER LIFE by Octavius Winslow, 1850

## US Food and Drug Administration

If Bittersweet (Atropine Belladonna) or Jimson Weed are used in some medications, they must be noted on the label the product contains them due to their poisonous actions. The plant Bittersweet (Atropine Belladonna) is considered an unsafe poisonous herb as it contains the alkaloid solanine.[85] Under 21 CFR 250.12, products containing Jimson weed are misbranded when the packaging contains directions for use in self-medication. If an over-the-counter cough medication contains Jimson Weed, which is a nightshade plant, it thus contains solanine and must receive approval according to the Federal Food Drug and Cosmetic Act, Section 102 (p).

The USDA is aware of the toxic nature of solanine; the problem is the nature of public acceptance. It remains unclear why the USDA has not alerted the public to the dangers of nightshades. Nor is it clear as to why the medical establishment is not eliminating nightshades as a possible source of many diseases, before starting expensive medical treatment.

---

[85] a-Chaconine [20562-03-2] and a-Solanine [20562-02-1],Review of Toxicological Literature, Prepared for Errol Zeiger, Ph.D., National Institute of Environmental Health Sciences

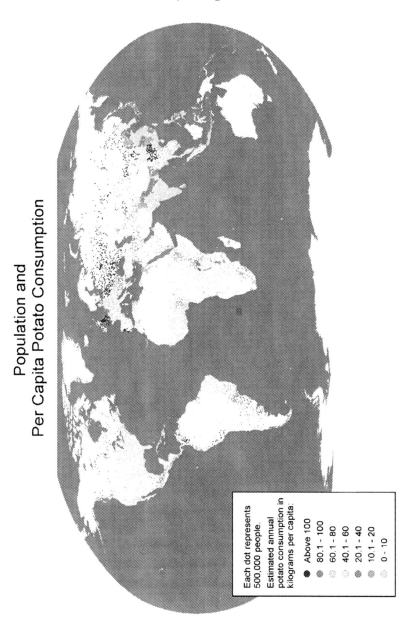

Population and
Per Capita Potato Consumption

Each dot represents 500,000 people.

Estimated annual potato consumption in kilograms per capita:

Above 100
80.1 - 100
60.1 - 80
40.1 - 60
20.1 - 40
10.1 - 20
0 - 10

Source: International Potato Center (CIP) 2006 used with permission
Heavy consumption is England. Please go to
http://research.cip.cgiar.org/confluence/display/wpa/Global+Maps
to see map in color.

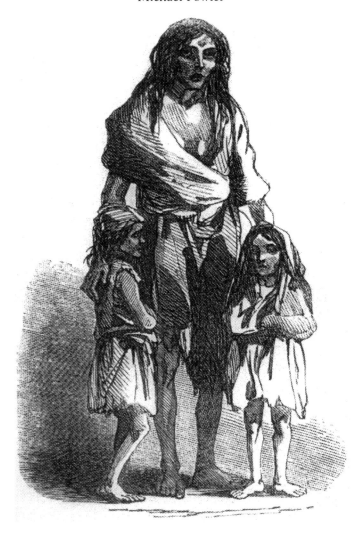

*Irish Family during the Famine*
*"You left us in tatters without shoes or socks, tired of digging potatoes, and spudding up docks; and now you've gay bracelets and bright feathers three! 'Yes: that how we dress when we're runied,' said she."*
-Thomas Hardy (1840-1928), British poet

# Part II: Nightshades and Health

## Safe Levels?

*"The Committee considered that, despite the long history of human consumption of plants containing glycoalkaloids, the available epidemiological and experimental data from human and laboratory animal studies did not permit the determination of a safe level of intake."* [86]

-Bureau of Chemical Safety Health and Welfare Canada

There have not been studies found on safe levels of nightshade plants. If there has been, they are not listed with the U.N. or Universities and the U.S. Government has never seen them. There are some studies done on the harmful levels of nightshades, but not the safe levels. People have thought nightshades were safe to eat because one million Irish can't be wrong. Well, they needed something to eat, because the British took all of their food. I would eat a potato rather than starve to death. When Sir Walter Raleigh introduced potatoes, no one did any studies to see if they might be harmful. People eat them and are not made immediately sick, so it was assumed, and still is, that nightshades are safe. In fact the way they came up with the level is by setting it just below the point when people start

---

[86] *SOLANINE AND CHACONINE:*First draft prepared by Dr T. Kuiper-Goodman and Dr P.S.Nawrot Bureau of Chemical Safety Health and Welfare Canada Ottawa, Ontario, Canada

to get sick. 2mg solanine/kg body weight, or 2mg/kg. This is same way the level of Vitamin C was set; people get scurvy at levels less than 40mg/day, so the current RDA is 50mg, just over the amount needed to prevent scurvy, but far lower than the body needs for other things such as immune system support.

Lewis and Clark were given mercury to ingest on their journey to the west coast, "to protect them from disease." Mercury is toxic. Solanine is toxic.

In 1907, an American pediatrician claimed that X-ray treatment could shrink the thymus of infants and prevent their death. This method continued to be used well into the next 50 years! Thankfully, it was stopped once researchers began to see a link between the growing number of cancer patients and their medical history that involved X-ray treatment.

Another "miracle" was introduced in the 1960s: a cholesterol reducing agent. Thought to be the ultimate cure for arteriosclerosis, it successfully became the agent for cataracts, hair loss, and impotence. There have been countless other mistakes, and oversights to match those.

Low-level long-term studies have not been done on the effects of nightshades on human beings. Neurology was an unknown science until 1921, when Sir Charles Sherrington discovered neurotransmitters. Many did not accept his theory at the time, but it proved to be true. Previously nerves were thought to be continuous or wire like and not a series of "switches." Sherrington believed that neurotransmission was purely electrical, later it was discovered that it is electrical and chemical. We now know that nightshade neurotoxins interfere with this process.

Eric Kandel who studied simple neural networks in sea-snails, *aplyisa*[87] discovered what he called *habituation*[88]. The snails have a gill reflex that causes them to withdraw if they are touched. Kandel would repeatedly touch the gills until the snails learned that stimulation was harmless, and

---

[87] The genus Aplysia belongs to the family Aplysiidae and is a genus of sea hares, which are a type of sea slug. The general description of these sea hares can be found under the entry about the superfamily Aplysioidea (Sea hares)

[88] habituation is an example of non-associative learning in which there is a progressive diminution of behavioral response probability with repetition of a stimulus. It is another form of integration. An animal first responds to a stimulus, but if it is neither rewarding nor harmful the animal reduces subsequent responses.

would no longer withdraw them. Significantly, it was learned by an automatic response system, not what we would generally consider a system that "learns." So what caused the change? Kandel discovered it was a change in the amount of neurotransmitters; each time he touched the gills less and less of the neurotransmitters was released.

By using the "habituation" method the reflex can be completely removed over time, and the neural pathways will degrade or disappear. The more you use a neural pathway the stronger it becomes, and the contrary is also true, that the less you use a neural pathway, the weaker it becomes. By constantly flooding, the nervous system with neurotoxins from nightshades on a daily basis we are challenging our entire system to function with reduced ability. As the stimulus is reduced introduction of neurotoxins, the entire nervous system becomes less effective. This should make the old anachronism, "use it or lose it," a little more relevant in our lives. Because that is exactly how the nervous system works, disuse eventually causes disappearance, and use causes improvement. This is why physical speed develops with repeated operations, the nerves slowly becoming stronger and faster with use and time

Nightshade plants can vary greatly in solanine content, and it accumulates in the body. These two facts make it unsafe as a staple food. If we ate potatoes just once a year, say on New Years Day, then it would be of no concern; however, we eat them every day.

The major neurotoxins contained in potatoes are as follows: Solanine, atropine, chaconine, nicotine, tomatine, scopolamine, and more. Each one affects humans in a different way. One of them, atropine, is a blocker preventing neurotransmission. The other three scopolamine, solanine, and chaconine, are powerful acetylcholinesterase inhibitors that prevent the breakdown of neurotransmitters need for proper nerve function.

We consume other kinds of neurotoxins, such as caffeine in coffee, tea, and sodas, and nicotine in tobacco, cocaine and others in legal and illegal drugs. Those neurotoxins are very different from solanine in nightshades, as they are water-soluble and leave your body quickly, generally within 24 hours. Solanine is not water-soluble; it stays in your body and is accumulated in the body organs.

The average American is ingesting about 13mg per day of solanine and it has a 1-2% excretion[89] rate per day. That means if you ingest 10mg on Tuesday, that only 0.2 mg will leave your body on Wednesday. Your body cannot convert solanine into anything else. It does not become a sugar, or fat; it always remains solanine. It lodges somewhere in the body, namely: the smooth muscles, abdominals and organs such as the intestines, heart, lungs, and the endocrine system, namely the thyroid.

*"Low rates of excretion were seen in urine and faeces[sic], and together accounted for about 5% of the administered dose during the first 24 h. Thus a fraction in excess of 90% of the dose was sequestered somewhere in the body 24 h after dosing. After this time, the rate of elimination from the body was low, about 1-2% per day, corresponding to an overall half-life of 34 to 68 days. The authors calculated that if absorption of solanine were 1 mg/day, then with a fractional rate of excretion of 0.02, the body burden would be 50 mg. The authors suggested that mobilization from various storage loci could occur during times of 'metabolic stress', including pregnancy (Claringbold et al., 1982)."*

We all understand the short-term effects of smoking, red eyes, coughing, dizziness, etc.; these are reduced after the person continues to smoke. We tend not to notice the long-term effects at first: cancer, emphysema, chronic coughing, and sometimes death.

All nightshade plants contain a neurotoxin that does not leave the body quickly; that neurotoxin is Solanine. The short-term effects of nightshade poisons can be very mild, such as sleepiness, and dizziness. For many people the effects are much more intense, such as chronic migraine headaches, dizziness, intestinal disturbance, and "food poisoning" like symptoms, which many people do not connect with nightshade plants such as potatoes.

The long-term problems of nightshade consumption are seen, but not connected with nightshades, i.e. cancer, I.B.S., joint problems, etc. Nightshade toxins attack the body in terms of cancer in at least four ways: one nicotine, which prevents the immune system from fighting cancer; two, solanine that interferes with the absorption of Vitamin $D_3$ needed to fight

---

[89] Excretion: The action of casting out of the body that which has been separated by any of the organs; esp. evacuation of the bowels.

cancer; three, disrupting cells, leading to potential susceptibility to cancers; Four, suppressing the endocrine system needed fight cancer.

Solanine leaches calcium from the bones, causes disturbances in the endocrine system, heart palpitations, and slight mental dysfunctions. The problem does not result from one or two exposures, but from a steady diet. Solanine accumulates in the body over years, and may be the leading cause of arthritis and other degenerative diseases. It can also be the cause of the misdiagnosis of Crohn's disease, or IBS (irritable bowel syndrome). All of this is described in part III of this book.

Most of us are aware that Tomatoes contain Lycopene, which was thought to prevent cancer. Recently the F.D.A. reported that there is *"no credible evidence"*[90] that this is the case. Potatoes contain vitamin C, and other beneficial items, however none of this can eliminate the toxic affects of Solanine. Just as if someone were to tell you that tobacco contained high amounts of vitamin C, you know this would not counter-balance the harmful effects of smoking. Nightshade plants are medicinal plants, which are a great benefit to us. Another example is the poppy(not a nightshade), which gives us opium for pain relief drugs. It was not until the early part of the 17th century that nightshades began to be eaten as a food at all, with the exception of the Inca Indians of Peru as potatoes are native to Peru.

The purpose of this book is not to frighten or cause a panic, it is simply to inform. The work of research has already been done on the effects of nightshades. What has not been done is adequately informing the public, which is the purpose of this book.

One last thing, many people will say, *"So what if you are allergic to potatoes, you certainly cannot claim they are bad for everyone!"* An allergy causes a histamine reaction in body. The body thinks that some chemical is a germ and it needs to be attacked, so it sends out histamine to rally the troops, so to speak, that will remove the intruder. This will give you watery eyes, runny nose, and such. The reactions people have to the neurotoxins found in nightshades are not a histamine reaction. In fact, potatoes are indeed an allergy-free food; that is why they are so popular in medicine. Rice is also an

---

[90] The U.S. Food and Drug Administration's Evidence-Based Review for Qualified Health Claims: *Tomatoes, Lycopene, and Cancer*: Claudine J. Kavanaugh, Paula R. Trumbo, Kathleen C. Ellwood; J Natl Cancer Inst, July 18, 2007; 99(14): 1060 - 1062.

allergy-free food, and contains no neurotoxins. The problems from night-shades are not allergic reaction; they are from the neurotoxins contained within.

Nightshades were introduced into the human diet long before any kind of testing for safety could be done. Modern tests have shown them to be unsafe, and dangerous as food stuffs. Yet, the public has not been made aware of these facts. Until now.

It is not currently easy to test nightshades for solanine concentrations; it is a long process that must be done in the lab. Simple field tests are not yet in available. A new potato variety was produced by traditional breeding methods that resulted in high levels of solanine. It was only after it went to market that concern was raised, and it has been withdrawn from public consumption. [91] What this means is the testing is only randomly done rather than systematically, as with items such as cow's milk which is test constantly. Another variable that must be considered is that potatoes will greatly increase in solanine content if exposed to light or bruised.

In a newsletter for perishables handling by Marita Cantwell, several concerns were raised. The first was the ease with which solanine could be quickly increased above the "generally accepted safe limits" of 20mg/100g (1/4 pound or one large health potato) of potato. There are more than 20 well-documented reports of human injury or death from the solanine poisoning from potatoes. [92] Due to variations in handling, the average content in the peelings can range from 3 to 100mg/100mg, and peeled potatoes can range from 0.10 mg to 4.5 mg/100mg. [93]

Solanine can increase in the dark, but that formation is only 20% of the rate of potatoes exposed to light. The rate of formation is dependent on the temperature as well; the rate doubles at 75°F as compared to 45°F. It is possible, in a well-lit and warm retail environment, for the solanine

---

[91] Biotechnology Overview, Product Applications, Consumer Response, Christine M. Bruhn, University of California, Davis

[92] Institute of Food Technologists, 2000

[93] A Review of Important Facts about Potato Glycoalkaloids, Perishables Handling Newsletter Issue No. 87, August 1996, page 26

content to reach 180 mg/100 g of peel.[94] This increase would not be detectable visually, and exceeds the accepted levels by <u>nine times</u>. Temporary gastrointestinal problems can occur from levels as low as 3-10mg/100g of potato.[95] In laboratory testing of humans and solanine, levels as low as 2mg/kg of human body weight have produced poisoning symptoms. Therefore, if a person who weighed 80kg were to eat 100g of potato peels at 180mg solanine, symptoms should occur. Symptoms from solanine poisoning can include headache, nausea, fatigue, vomiting, abdominal pain and cramps, and diarrhea.

Cooking does not reduce the solanine content, unless cooked to temperatures above 470°F[96] throughout, which results in rather unpleasant potatoes.

Another concern is that if potatoes are not "hilled" properly, meaning covered with dirt while growing, they can be exposed to sunlight which will increase the solanine content.[97] This concern had greatly increased as nearly all commercially grown potatoes are cultivated mechanically.

Solanine content per 100 gram serving:[98]

- Common Peppers          7.7-9.2
- Eggplant                6.1-11.33
- Potatoes                2-13

---

[94] A Review of Important Facts about Potato Glycoalkaloids, Perishables Handling Newsletter Issue No. 87, August 1996, page 26

[95] Ibid

[96] a-Chaconine [20562-03-2] and a-Solanine [20562-02-1],Review of Toxicological Literature, Prepared for Errol Zeiger, Ph.D., National Institute of Environmental Health Sciences

[97] University of Purdue HORT410 - Vegetable Crops

[98] Childers N.F. A relationship of arthritis to the Solanaceae (nightshades). J Intern Acad Prev Med 1979; 7:31-37

## Nicotine in Nightshades (Smoking Taters)

Nicotine is found in the following amount in nightshades plants and in Cauliflower[99], which is not part of the nightshade family. Eggplant is of far higher content than all others.[100] 174g serving of Eggplant would deliver 15ug. What is 15ug? Well a common cigarette delivers about 1.5 mg(milligrams) of nicotine to the smoker[101]. 15ug is the same as 0.015 mg so not much per serving.

The average nightshade eater will consume about one cigarettes worth of nicotine every two weeks. That amount by any standard is very low. Of course, one might ask how much nicotine its take to get cancer? At this point, some people will say "big deal." Here is the scary part if you sit in a room for 3 hours with a smoker you will absorb 1ug of nicotine. Secondhand smoke causes approximately 3,400 lung cancer deaths and 22,700-69,600 heart disease deaths in adult nonsmokers in the United States each year.[102] Secondhand smoke is responsible for between 150,000 and 300,000 lower respiratory tract infections in infants and children under 18 months of age, resulting in between 7,500 and 15,000 hospitalizations each year, and causes 1,900 to 2,700 sudden infant death syndrome (SIDS) deaths in the United States annually.[103]

The study by Domino et al[104] stated that someone eating 10g of eggplant or 244g of tomato would be the same as spending three hours in a room lightly polluted with cigarette smoke. Second-hand smoke has been

---

[99] Due the low consumption of cauliflower and the lack of other toxins that are present in nightshades, it seems unnecessary to raise an alert to the use of cauliflower, but some may wish to exclude it.

[100] The New England Journal of Medicine Volume 329:437 August 5, 1993 Number 6 : *The Nicotine Content of Common Vegetables*, by Edward F. Domion, M.D. Erich Hornback, B.A., Tsenge Demana, Ph.D.

[101] Hukkanen, J., Jacob, P. III, Benowitz, N. L. (2005). *Metabolism and Disposition Kinetics of Nicotine*. Pharmacol. Rev. 57: 79-115

[102] California Environmental Protection Agency. *Health Effects of Exposure to Environmental Tobacco Smoke*. June 2005.

[103] Ilib.

[104] Domino EF, Hornbach E, Demana T. *The nicotine content of common vegetables*. N Engl J Med 1993;329:437.

proven to be so toxic to bystanders that smoking indoors or in the work place has been banned by most states, yet not a peep of information appears on the effects of nightshade plants in the diet.

Nicotine can be broken down in the body into byproducts cotinine and nicotine-N-oxide. Solanine has not been found to break down by any of the body's processes.

In fact, if you wanted to you could smoke potato, tomato, or egg-plant leaves. You could also eat tobacco tubers. The point is that nicotine is in all nightshades and has dangerous effects: ". . . *there is a wealth of observations proving that nicotine has many actions on the central nervous system. In the brain as in the periphery, small doses of nicotine tend to stimulate functions which are blocked by higher doses. . . . Condition reflexes have been inhibited in . . . Nicotine in fairly high doses causes desynchronization in the electro-encephalogram. In sufficiently large doses typical [epileptic] 'grand mal' seizure patterns appear. Tremor is a result of central stimulation by nicotine," p 932. "In toxic doses, nicotine blocks parasympathetic ganglia," p 931.)* [105]

---

[105] W. Kalow, M.D., *Some Aspects of the Pharmacology of Nicotine* 4 Applied Therapeutics (#10) 930-932 (Oct 1962)

| Vegetable | Highest Reported Mean Nicotine Content | Reference | Amount of Vegetable Required to Obtain 1 μg of Nicotine* |
|---|---|---|---|
| | ng/g | | g |
| Cauliflower | 16.8 | Davis et al.[4] | 59.5 |
| Cauliflower | 3.8 | Present study | 263.4 |
| Eggplant | 100.0 | Castro and Monji[2] | 10.0 |
| Potato peel | 4.8 | Davis et al.[4] | 208.0 |
| Potato pulp | 15.3 | Davis et al.[4] | 65.4 |
| Potatoes | 7.1 | Present study | 140.4 |
| Green tomatoes | 42.8 | Castro and Monji[2] | 23.4 |
| Pureed tomatoes | 52.0 | Castro and Monji[2] | 19.2 |
| Ripe tomatoes | 4.3 | Castro and Monji[2] | 233.0 |
| Ripe tomatoes | 4.1 | Present study | 244.0 |
| Tomatoes | 10.7 | Sheen[3] | 93.5 |

*One microgram of nicotine is the amount a passive smoker would absorb in about three hours in a room with a minimal amount of tobacco smoke.

The New England Journal of Medicine, Volume 329:437 August 5, 1993

## USDA table of Nutrients for Potatoes

In the USDA's database there are 149 items on potatoes, but nothing on solanine, atropine, potatoes with green skin, or anything else that might suggest any kind of danger. You would think the amount of nicotine and solanine would at least be as important as the amount of *ash* in the potato. I mean who cares about ash?

*Potatoes, baked, skin, without salt*   NDB No:   11364

| Nutrient | Units | Value per 100 grams of edible portion | Sample Count | Std. Error | 1 skin ‾‾‾ 58 g |
|---|---|---|---|---|---|
| **Proximates** | | | | | |
| Water | g | 47.31 | 6 | 1.891 | 27.440 |
| Energy | kcal | 198 | 0 | | 114.840 |
| Energy | kj | 830 | 0 | | 481.400 |
| Protein | g | 4.29 | 4 | 0.270 | 2.488 |
| Total lipid (fat) | g | 0.10 | 0 | | 0.058 |
| Ash | g | 2.24 | 4 | 0.115 | 1.299 |
| Carbohydrate, by difference | g | 46.06 | 0 | | 26.715 |
| Fiber, total dietary | g | 7.9 | 0 | | 4.582 |
| Sugars, total | g | 1.40 | 0 | | 0.812 |
| **Minerals** | | | | | |
| Calcium, Ca | mg | 34 | 6 | 9.770 | 19.720 |
| Iron, Fe | mg | 7.04 | 6 | 1.901 | 4.083 |
| Magnesium, Mg | mg | 43 | 6 | 1.960 | 24.940 |

USDA National Nutrient Database for Standard Reference, Release 16 (July 2003)

One report states that 387 smoker mental disorder symptoms including "*rebellion*" and "*a considerable feeling of defiance for authority and the individuating thrill of setting aside some rule.*" and "*Clinical experimental data indicate that a definite physiologic addiction to nicotine exists,*" and "*indicating pharmacologic addiction to nicotine.*"[106]

"*The long-term brain changes observed among cocaine and heroin users can also be found in the brains of smokers, researchers from the National Institute on*

[106] Barry, Maurice J., Jr., M.D., *Psychologic Aspects of Smoking*, 35 Staff Meetings of Mayo Clinic (#13) 386 (22 June 1960)

*Drug Abuse (NIDA) say. . . . changes to smokers' brains could be observed even years after they quit . . . abnormally high levels of a pair of enzymes involved in the dopamine system . . . changes . . . the same among smokers as among other drug users... The fact that the changes were the same among smokers as among other drug users "strongly suggests" that they contribute to addiction, said Hope."[107]*

## Neurology 101

First, it is necessary to talk about neurology, before talking about neurotoxins [108]such as solanine[109]. According to people who know these things, there are estimated to be 100 billion nerves cells in our bodies. That is about the same number as stars in the Milky Way galaxy. For every nerve cell, there are about 1000 other nerve cells that can send it information. That nerve cell in turn can send information to about the same number. This makes computers look like small potatoes.

The result is that we cannot understand the nervous system–it is far to complex. We can only identify some of the parts, and actions the make up the nervous system. Phenomena such as memory, thoughts, emotions, responses, senses, are completely unknown in there origins. The nervous system is massive communications system. What is incredible is that the information sent performs tasks. When the brain sends a signal to the hand the hand does not process the information, it responds–a true marvel.

Most people understand that the nerves in our bodies send electrical signals back and forth, which allows our body's parts to communicate with other parts. We have sensors in our skin that tell us when we feel hot or cold, soft or hard, fuzzy or smooth, etc.

When our eye receives light from outside sources, tiny electrical signals are sent to our brain that construct a visual image of the world around

---

[107] Bruce Hope, et al., *Nicotine, Other Drugs Have Similar Brain Effects* Journal of Neuroscience, 21 February 2007
[108]Neurotoxin: a substance having a poisonous effect on the nerves
[109] Solanine: A poisonous alkaloid, or a compound containing an alkaloid, found in various plants of the genus Solanum

us. Transmitting all this information is done by the nervous system. Nerves are both chemical and electrical in their function.

When a nerve is stimulated, an electrical potential is created that sends an electrical pulse down to the end of the nerve. When the electrical pulse reaches the end of the nerve it activates small chemical transmitters.

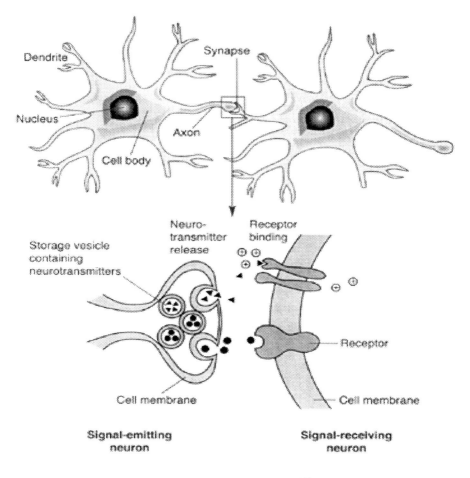

*Nerve cells and synapse* [110]

---

[110] Goodlett, C.R., and Horn, K.H. *Mechanisms of alcohol-induced damage to the developing nervous system.* Alcohol Research & Health 25(3):175–184, 2001

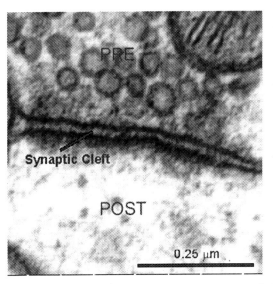

These transmitters discharge a chemical called a neurotransmitter [111]that traverses a small gap called the synapse[112].

On the other side of this gap is another nerve which receives those neuro-transmitters and causes that nerve to be stimulated.

*Image: synapse, viewed with an electron microscope[113]*

If enough neurotransmitters are delivered then the next nerve cell in the chain will fire. We see a chain reaction from electrical to chemical and from chemical to electrical. That is the simple version. See Figure 1. Neurotransmission.

In Figure 1 (A) is the transmitter area of the neuron. When the neuron (A) is stimulated it releases a neurotransmitter (7) called acetylcholine[114]. It is this neurotransmitter's job to traverse the gap from one nerve to the other. The gap or synapse(4) is so small that it is barely observable with an electron microscope, so the little neurotransmitters do not have far to go. On the other side of the gap is the postsynaptic receptor (B). It contains little areas called neural receivers (5) that receive a neurotransmit-

---

[111] Neurotransmitter: A substance which is released at the end of a nerve fibre by the arrival of a nerve impulse and, by diffusing across the synapse or junction, effects the transfer of the impulse to another nerve fibre, a muscle fibre, or some other receptor.
[112] Synapse: The junction, or structure at the junction, between two neurons or nerve-cells
[113] Synapse Web, Kristen M. Harris, PI; Copyright © Synapse Web 1999-2007
[114] Acetylcholine: The acetyl ester of choline, C7H17O3N, a chemical secreted at the ends of many nerve-fibres.

ter. The presynaptic area is (7) before the gap (synapse), the postsynaptic area is (5) after the gap (synapse).

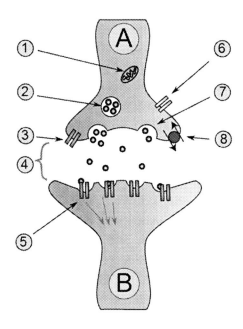

**Figure 1 Neurotransmission by Fr. Utilisateur**

A : Neuron (Presynaptic)
B : Neuron (Postsynaptic)
1. Mitochondria
2. Synaptic vesicle full of neurotransmitter
3. Autoreceptor
4. Synaptic cleft
5. Neurotransmitter receptor
6. Calcium Channel
7. Fused vesicle releasing neurotransmitter
8. Neurotransmitter reuptake pump

Once the neurotransmitters are received the nerve is stimulated into action, if a sufficient amount of neurotransmitters have been delivered (that is what those little arrows in (B) are trying to show). There is what is called a threshold limit in the nervous system. That means unless a certain amount of neurotransmitters are delivered, nothing happens. A small amount of neurotransmitter delivery, does <u>not result</u> in a small amount of information being conveyed, rather it results in <u>no information</u> being conveyed. This is called *the all or nothing effect*. What does this mean to you and I? If we are running low on neurotransmitters, (lack of sleep, poor diet, etc) then we lose the ability to transmit information, which means the ability to think clearly or quickly. The more neurotransmitters we have the quicker and easier it is to think. Caffeine in coffee excites the release of neurotransmitters, so we can think better, but at a cost, as we run out quicker.

Once the acetylcholine (neurotransmitter) has jumped the synapse (gap) and contacted the postsynaptic receptor (receiver), and the nerve has fired, its job is done. If the neurotransmitter remains lodged in the postsynaptic receptor forever, that nerve can never operate again. As it is being blocked by the neurotransmitter, that neurotransmitter can no longer stimulate the nerve to fire.

To prevent this from happening there is an enzyme in the body called Acetylcholinesterase.[115] This enzyme has an extremely important function; when it comes in contact with the neurotransmitter acetylcholine it causes that neurotransmitter to break down into its component parts, acetyl and choline. Once a neurotransmitter has been broken apart, it then leaves the neuroreceptor and is reabsorbed into the presynaptic neuron to be used again. (8) This allows the neuroreceptor to receive new information should it be delivered. To get an idea of how fast this operates, the enzyme Acetylcholinesterase can break down 10,000 neurotransmitters per second. Please understand, all of this is an oversimplification of many possible processes that would be overwhelming for this book.

Now we are going to talk about neurodysfunctions. This is where neurotoxins come in. If a chemical prevents any of the operations in neurotransmission from functioning, it is known as a neurotoxin. The first kind of neurotoxin is one that affects the receptor. By affecting the receptor it stops the neurotransmitter from uniting with the receptor and causing electro-stimulation, which will in turn prevent communication in the nervous system.

---

[115]Acetylcholinesterase: A cholinesterase that causes rapid hydrolysis of acetylcholine after the transmission of a nerve impulse.

This can be wanted or unwanted as the case may be. Example: If someone is in extreme pain, we may want to "deaden" the nerves to give comfort to the person. The neurotoxin atropine affects postsynaptic receptors, by blocking the reception areas on the neuron. This means that when the presynapitic neuron fires the neurotransmitters, those neuro-transmitters are not allowed to contact the receptor in order to convey information. Thus, the nerves telling you that you have stepped on a nail are no longer able to send a signal to your brain that this has happened, thus you can rest and sleep, rather then writhe in pain all night.

The next kind of neurotoxin does not affect the reception area but affects Acetylcholinesterase. Solanine is the neurotoxin that binds with this enzyme Acetylcholinesterase. The upshot is that the neurotransmitters are not removed from the neuroreceiver and thus there is a flooding of neuro-transmitters. This is how nerve gas works in chemical warfare. Most of the body's Acetylcholinesterase is bound up by the nerve agent and can no longer affect the neurotransmitters properly. When this happens all of the glands and nervous system become highly activated and eventually cause death by severe cramping and flooding of the body with all kinds of unnec-essary glandular secretions. It is truly a ghastly death.

Solanine affects the body the same way nerve gas does, just in a far less severe way. However, if a person were to ingest enough solanine it would have the same deadly effect. This is why solanine has become a cheap source of rat poison. [116]

The two effects of neurotoxins that we are concerned with are the prevention of reception, by blockers such as atropine or the prevention of disconnection of neurotransmitters by binding the enzyme Acetylcholi-nesterase.

Solanine in nightshades binds to the enzyme Acetylcholinesterase, and prevents it from removing neurotransmitters from the neuroreceptors.

---

[116] Journal of Neurological and Orthopedic Medical Surgery (1993) 12:227-231 *An Apparent Relation of Nightshades (Solanaceae) to Arthritis* N.F. Childers, Ph.D., and M.S. Margoles, M.D.

Atropine in nightshades binds to the neuroreceptors, and blocks neuro-transmission. This excess of acetylcholine generally causes "happy feelings", which can cause cravings for nightshades, this is the beginning of addiction. Then after the acethlcholine is used up, the person may experience a "crash," a.k.a. mood swings. Many people become sleepy from a lack of acetylcholine, as only sleep can restore them to the neurotransmitters.

Please also read the section on nightshades and Nerve Gas for more explanations.

## The Neurotoxins of Nightshades

### Atropine

Atropine is commonly used to treat asthma, brachicardia (abnormal heart beat), gastric ulcer treatment, hay fever, to slow the tremors caused by Parkinson's disease, and even by the United States government as an antidote for poisonous gas. Atropine that is manufactured synthetically can be utilized in surgery to stop fluids prior to surgery, and is used in nasal decongestants.

The alkaloid Atropine in the drug form "Atropine Sulphate" or "Sal-Tropine"[117] has a range of modern medical applications, but its roots originate in folklore. It is said that the witches of ancient Europe (circa. 1500 BC) used the plant in their "brews" to enable a person to fly. It was applied by rubbing on the body's "pulse points" on the hands, genitalia and feet. The drug is a derivative of tropine, a tropane alkaloid[118] like cocaine.[119] Tropines are a large chemical chain from which many drugs can be derived.

---

[117]*Evaluation of antidotes for poisoning by organophosphorus pesticides* Authors: Johnson, M.K.; Jacobsen, D.; Meredith, T.J.; Eyer, P.; Heath, A.J.; Ligtenstein, D.A.; Marrs, T.C.; Szinicz, L.; Vale, J.A.; Haines, J.A.Source: Emergency Medicine, Volume 12, Number 1, 1 March 2000 , pp. 22-37(16)Publisher: Blackwell Publishing

[118]A saturated bicyclic tertiary amine which is a basic liquid obtained from various plants and the parent of a series of compounds which includes atropine, cocaine, and related alkaloids; 8-methyl-8-azabicyclo-[3.2.1]octane, $C_8H_{15}N$.

[119] Cocaine: An important alkaloid obtained from the leaves and young twigs of the coca plant, valuable as a local anæsthesiant, and also used as a stuimulant.

Atropine begins to take effect 30-60 minutes after consumption and may last as much as 24-48 hours as these alkaloids repress the digestive tract (it is excreted in urine). It has a half-life of 2-3 days. After absorption from the gastro-intestinal tract, Atropine can increase the heart rate by a speed of 20 to 40 beats per minute, causes inhibition of secretions from glands, hence making dryness in the mouth, nose and then skin, and relaxes the intestinal muscles. It will also cross into the Central Nervous System (CNS) from the blood to the brain (through the Blood-Brain Barrier) and hence depresses and excites different parts of the CNS. It does this by interrupting the nerve receptors, acting as a "sympathetic cholinergic blocking agent," a blocking agent to the nerve transmitter acetylcholine. This effect is very prevalent in the elderly, inducing amnesia, excitation and mental confusion. It will also result in pupil dilation and an increase of pressure within the eye (intraocular pressure) with blurred vision. [120]

### Solanine

Solanine, a naturally occurring toxin found in nightshade plants is a non-water soluble chemical that is not destroyed by cooking. It can be reduced slightly by deep-frying at high temperatures, 470°F, but not completely. It is a stable, powerful cholinesterase inhibitor, an enzyme which affords agility of muscle movement. Solanine can cause muscle pain and spasms, joint pain and swelling, gastrointestinal disturbances, anorexia, nausea, vomiting and feelings of nervousness.

The anesthetic properties of tropane alkaloids may relate to their interference with acetylcholine, perhaps by competing with it at the synaptic junctions, thus blocking or inhibiting nerve impulses. It is interesting to note that the infamous tropane alkaloid, cocaine, is also a local anesthetic when injected into skin or muscle tissue. This probably led to the discovery

---

[120]*Evaluation of antidotes for poisoning by organophosphorus pesticides* Authors: Johnson, M.K.; Jacobsen, D.; Meredith, T.J.; Eyer, P.; Heath, A.J.; Ligtenstein, D.A.; Marrs, T.C.; Szinicz, L.; Vale, J.A.; Haines, J.A.Source: Emergency Medicine, Volume 12, Number 1, 1 March 2000 , pp. 22-37(16)Publisher: Blackwell Publishing

and synthesis of the more potent compound, Novocain[121], widely used in dentistry.

Organophosphate insecticides, such as Malathion and Parathion[122], bind to active sites on this enzyme, thus preventing the normal shut down of nerve impulses and destroying the nervous control of insects. Nerve gasses developed during World War II have a similar effect on the nervous system. Gulf War soldiers carried an atropine syrette to counter the possible effects of nerve gas.

If ingested in sufficient quantities, cardiac glycosides can be fatal by literally stopping the heart muscle.[123] What happens is that the nerves that control the heart become activated, and the heart muscle compresses and will not uncompress, thus it fails to pump blood, which leads to death.

## Cornell University (Veterinary Dept.)

*"Some fat-soluble plant toxins even bioaccumulate- that is, when an animal eats the plant, the toxins collect in animal tissues and pass to humans when we eat the animal and can be secreted in human and animal milk (for example, solanine from potatoes). Toxin concentrations in a plant can vary tremendously, often by 100X or more, and can be dramatically affected by environmental stress on the plant (drought, heat/cold, mineral deficiencies, etc) and disease. "*[124]

This raises even more concerns due to the fact that nightshades fed to animals are not regulated by the FDA.

---

[121] Novocain: used as a local anesthetic.
[122] An organophosphorus insecticides which are relatively harmless to plants and animals; in commercial preparations it is a brownish liquid with a strong smell of garlic and is also used in the form of a powder.
[123] Armstrong, W.P, Ph.D. 2001. Wayne's Word: 9 May 2001. http://waynesword.palomar.edu/wayne.htm (12 June 2001).
[124] Cornell University (Veterinary Dept.)

## Scopolamine

Scopolamine (skoh - pahl' - uh - meen), is derived from the bella-donna plant, and acts as an anticholinergic (that is, it interferes with acetylcholine, the chemical that allows nerves to fire), preventing nerves from working properly. In large doses it is extremely toxic, severely lower-ing the activity of nerves in the autonomic nervous system (the part of the nervous system that controls involuntary activity, like gland activity or cardiac muscle movement). Its main medical uses are related to its "anti-spasmodic" action, and include

- As a sedative given before anesthetic
- As a treatment for the tremors of Parkinson's Disease
- To dilate the pupils
- Reduce secretions from the sweat glands
- To prevent motion sickness

The scopolamine is absorbed into the body through the skin. It is not clear how scopolamine prevents nausea and vomiting due to motion sickness. The vestibular part of the ear is very important for balance. When a person becomes disoriented due to motion, the vestibule sends a signal through nerves to the vomiting center in the brain, and vomiting occurs. Acetylcholine is the chemical that nerves use to transmit messages to each other. Scientists believe that scopolamine prevents communication between the nerves of the vestibule and the vomiting center in the brain by blocking the action of acetylcholine. Scopolamine also may work directly on the vomiting center. Scopolamine must be taken before the onset of motion sickness to be effective.

## Nicotine

The most commonly known of all neurotoxins and is most preva-lent in the nightshade plant tobacco. Nicotine has powerful pharmacologic effects (including increased heart rate, heart stroke volume, and oxygen consumption by the heart muscle) as well as powerful psychodynamic effects (such as euphoria, increased alertness, and a sense of relaxation)

Nicotine is an agonist[125] that binds with the same neuro-receptors that acetylcholine does. This does two things, first it blocks acetylcholine from being received, thus it interferes with proper neruo-transmission, and it simulates the nerve cell that receives it in a way that acetylcholine does not. This is one of the reasons it is able to give a calming feeling to the smoker. Nicotine also causes the release of other neuro-transmitters that affect mood, appetite, and memory. Dopamine is one of these, very useful for the ability to think, especially for problem solving thinking. Dopamine also stimulates the pleasure center of the brain, gives the "rush" or "high" of smoking. This "rush" is what reinforces the desire for smoking. All three of the foregoing reasons are why people smoke when under stress; it calms them down, gives pleasure, and releases dopamine which allows the person to think about the problems that are stressing them in the first place.

These same factors are what cause the "withdrawal symptoms" when people quit smoking. Increase in stress, inability to think clearly, depression, increase in hunger, restlessness,

All nightshades contain nicotine, yes the potato, tomato, pepper, ect. contain the carcinogen. The levels are lower than in tobacco. Thus, you can make potato leaf cigarettes.

The body's nervous system adapts to the use of nicotine over time which is why it takes a greater amount of the drug to get the "rush" or effect after long-term use. It is this adaptation that leads to heavy smoking and addiction. The same kind of studies have not been done for solanine.

## Cooking

One of the more common myths about nightshade plants is the idea that cooking destroys solanine. "...*solanine: Heat-stable toxic compound (a glycoside of the alkaloid solanidine)*"[126]

---

[125] Agonist: A chemical which can not only combine with a neuro-receptor, like an antagonist, but when it does so stimulates it, resulting in an observable effect
[126] David A. Bender. *Solanine*, A Dictionary of Food and Nutrition, January 1, 2005.

*"Boiling is **not effective** in decreasing the concentrations of chaconine and solanine in potatoes (Takagi et al., 1990). Microwaving reduced the alkaloid content by 15%, and deep frying showed mixed results depending on cooking temperature. The authors noted that the critical temperature for the decomposition of both alkaloids in cooked potatoes was 170°C(470°F). Freeze drying and dehydration of potatoes reduced the glycoalkaloid content either slightly or not at all (Brain and Turner, 1971; Zaletskaya et al., 1977; both cited by Morris and Lee, 1984)."* [127]

It must be noted that potatoes are often baked at temperatures around 470°F, however the inside of the potato does not reach this temperature. For the solanine to begin to break down the entire potato must reach the temperature of 470° F, which would render it inedible.

## Peeling

Most of the solanine is contained in the peels of potatoes, but this can vary greatly. Although peeling will reduce the overall content of solanine and other alkaloids in potatoes, it will not eliminate them.

*"Thirty to eighty percent of the glycoalkaloids in the potato tuber are found in the outer layers (Meyer, 1895; Bomer and Mattis, 1924; Griebel, 1924; Wolf and Duggar, 1946; all cited by Maga, 1980). Thus, peeling generally reduces glycoalkaloid intake (Lagolo et al., 1991; cited by Hoskins, 1994). However, a study by Mondy and Gosselin (1988; cited by Beier, 1990) **concluded that peeling potatoes prior to cooking did not** decrease the glycoalkaloid content."* [128]

---

[127] a-Chaconine [20562-03-2] and a-Solanine [20562-02-1] Review of Toxicological Literature, Prepared for Errol Zeiger, Ph.D.,National Institute of Environmental Health Sciences,Submitted by Raymond Tice, Ph.D. ,Integrated Laboratory Systems,February 1998
[128] a-Chaconine [20562-03-2] and a-Solanine [20562-02-1] Review of Toxicological Literature, Prepared for Errol Zeiger, Ph.D.,National Institute of Environmental Health Sciences,Submitted by Raymond Tice, Ph.D. ,Integrated Laboratory Systems,February 1998

"*Fried potato peels are a source of large quantities of -chaconine and -solanine; one study indicated that fried potato peels had -chaconine plus -solanine levels of 1.4 to 1.5 mg/g potato peel (Bushway and Ponnampalam, 1981), which is* **seven times the recommended upper** *safety* **limit** (0.2 mg/g potato) (Beier, 1990)." [129]


## Potato Fungus

As a side note, since we are talking about potatoes and health problems related to them, recently a fungus has been found on potatoes with dry-rot, and it is deadly: "*Rotting potatoes harbor harmful toxins Shriveled brown spots on potatoes may indicate deadly trichothecene toxins. a new study suggests that potentially harmful levels of the poisons may occur in potatoes infected with a major fungal perpetrator of potato dry-rot, says coauthor Anne E. Desjardins, a biochemist at USDA's Agricultural Research Service in Peoria, Ill. If a careful survey of store-bought potatoes confirms these preliminary findings, the safety of infected potatoes 'may be something to think about,' Desjardins says. However, she emphasizes that it is unclear how much harm the toxin levels found in the study would cause in humans. 'There's routine screening for toxins in corn and wheat ... but potato farmers have never really thought about it,'*"[130]

She goes on to say that the fungus is heat stable so cooking will not destroy it, nor will trimming remove all of the toxins. The fungus can grow in as little as six days in the right conditions.

The effects of the toxins can range form vomiting and hair loss to immunosuppression, central nervous system dysfunction, coma and death, according to Desjardins.[131]

---

[129] Ibid
[130] *Rotting potatoes harbor harmful toxins.* (Food Science), Science News, April 15, 1989.
[131] Ibid

# Pets and Potatoes

Nightshades have been a troublesome pasture plant for owners of livestock for centuries. Normally, animals will avoid nightshades unless starving; sometimes horses will browse upon nightshade plants due to boredom. Until recently, it has been very rare for dogs and cats to have any contact with nightshades, as they will not naturally eat them.

However, recently food companies and veterinarians who seem to have forgotten the lessons learned with livestock are now suggesting and introducing nightshades in the diets of dogs and cats. Nightshades are highly poisonous to dogs and cats. In fact, the only two animals that are known to be able to tolerate nightshades at all of are rabbits and goats, but even they will be killed by Jimson Weed, or Potato leaves.

Recently, my neighbor took their dog to the veterinarian because it had a skin problem. One of the things the veterinarian recommended was giving the dog some slices of potato during the day, as potatoes are an allergy free food, she was asked why is it that potatoes are harmful to horses, which are vegetarian animals, and yet you are suggesting them for a dog which is a carnivore. After some stumbling upon her words, she gave no good reasons other than she did not think they would be harmful.

An article that I recently read on a web site about cats was talking about a similar incident that they had with their veterinarian and nightshades. However odd it might be for a cat to eat a cherry tomato, they had one that did. They reported about 100g fresh organic cherry tomato that "Kitty," for some reason, gobbled down. 100g is about 5 ounces, or about three small cherry tomatoes, which seems like quite a bit for a cat. Not knowing how poisonous solanine is to felines, they did not induce vomiting to purge the cat. The next day the cat committed "perjury", without any help. It did this about every three to four hours; the cat was clearly out of order.

When they asked the veterinarian about it, they said it was "dietary indiscretion," not to worry. Even though the cat continued eating, he would vomit up his meal within about an hour. After 48 hours it refused to eat, would only drink water; the vomiting continued and now vigorous diarrhea started. The cat became lethargic and withdrew; a trip to the veterinary office ruled out an intestinal blockage or an infection, however, Kitty was severely dehydrated. The cat's breathing was labored and rapid, his movement was slow and he had trembling of limbs. This continued on to day five, when it was clear that their cat was dying. A second veterinarian began to treat for poisoning, at which point the cat's health improved after six days. She went on to say that after two weeks the cat was still recovering from its tomato poisoning. This is from the web site called *Cats of Feline Future, by Natasha Will.*

She was kind enough to post a statement from the Cornell book of cats on poisoning.

The Cornell Book of Cats 2nd edition adapted from p. 383 Reference Guide: First Aid for Plant Poisoning:

*Vomiting, abdominal pain, bloody diarrhea, dry mouth, all after a latent period of 18-24 hours after plant was eaten. May proceed to nervous system stimulation followed by, i.e., trembling, salivation, and paralysis. May lead to cardiac arrest.*

*Common Plants: Nightshades, Jerusalem cherry, Potato (green parts and eyes).*

*Treatment : Induce vomiting if possible, but exercise caution: the gastrointestinal tract may already have suffered extensive damage that vomiting would exacerbate. Get the cat to your veterinarian promptly so that he or she can provide the necessary supportive therapy.*

I copied an article from the Washington Post, produced by Dr. Fox, to show the relative ignorance of modern veterinarians in terms of nightshade plants. Dr. Fox believes that only green sprouting potatoes contain solanine, therefore potatoes are perfectly fine in a dog's diet. Of all the things in the world that dogs can eat, I would not think it is necessary to push any boundaries of sensibilities and feed them nightshades.

Of even greater concern to me is that so many pet foods are now being produced with potatoes as a base, namely because they are cheap. I would certainly avoid feeding my pets any food that contains nightshades. You will see that Dr. Fox attributed the dog's vomiting to an allergic reaction to the potatoes not to their poisonous nature. Dogs will not naturally eat potatoes; they will only eat them if their master serves them— sometimes.

*Dear Dr. Fox:*
*In one of your columns, a reader mentioned that her veterinarian had prescribed*

*a "potato-based diet." Recently I read a book by a veterinarian who stated that the potato is "poison to a dog." Who is right? When I gave my own dog a potato-based stew, she promptly vomited the potato bits in it. I now carefully check ingredients in my dog food. Please comment.*

*G.J., Silver Spring*

*The potato is a highly nutritious vegetable that is not normally poisonous to dogs. Many experienced veterinarians and animal nutritionists recommend including potato in home-prepared dog food. However, potatoes that have turned green and are sprouting can be toxic. They are related, like the tomato, to the deadly Nightshade, the poison called solanine. So no one should eat old sprouting spuds or feed them to their dogs or pigs! As for your dog's experience with a potato-based stew, other ingredients in it might have caused an **allergic reaction or indigestion.**[132]*

No, Dr. Fox, it is the toxin solanine that is not good for dogs or people. Of course, you have to love a veterinarian named Dr. Fox.

## A Nightshade Diet

If one were to continue to ingest nightshades, it would seem logical to do so in the following manner. Potatoes that are not green, bruised, or rotten, should be carefully peeled to remove as much of the solanine as possible. Nightshades should not be used as a staple food, but used only on occasion, to reduce the total amount of solanine ingested. Children, the elderly, and hopeful, expecting, or nursing mothers, should completely avoid them.

The solanine content is markedly reduced in tomatoes when they are vine ripened, which is not the case for commercially grown, or store bought. As the tomato ripens solanine is converted to sugar, which is why vine ripened tomatoes are sweetest, however, they still contain considerable amounts of solanine. Please review the chart in *Nicotine in Nightshades*

---

[132] Animal Doctor, Dear Dr. Fox, The Washington Post, August 7, 2001.

(*Smoking Taters*) to see the difference between vine ripened and green tomatoes. Store bought tomatoes are harvested green, then ripened in warehouses; this does not ripen them properly, which is why vine ripened are so much sweeter. I am only suggesting this action for people who find it impossible to completely eliminate nightshades from their diet. I for one will never eat them again, save famine.

## Detoxifying

When I speak of detoxifying it is not a reference to acute poisoning; in such cases seek immediate medical aid.

This is a short chapter on how to remove solanine from the body that has accumulated over the years. This will happen naturally over time; most studies or experts say that the first stage of nightshade alkaloid will leave the body in 24-48 hours. There are detoxifying teas and systems available on the market. However, they are considered ineffective by most at doing anything other then help you pass a drug test, so save your money.

Second stage, getting built up alkaloids out of your system: time is probably the easiest way. Most conclude that it takes about two or three months to eliminate the majority of alkaloids from your system, as they are stored in fat and other tissues, but there are not any good studies on this. Some suggest drinking acidic drinks like citrus, orange juice, grapefruit juice and such, as the acids will bond with the alkaloids; who knows how effective overall this will be, but it cannot hurt. Exercise will help move out toxins of all kinds.

Dieting will drain fat reserves which may release stored alkaloids, so you might feel some effects, but it will be temporary. As always, drink lots of pure water.

Many people find that after a detoxifying period they can return to eating nightshades; this is true but the bad effects will return.

# Part III: Symptoms and Effects of Night-shades

## Possible Short Term Effects

Effects on the nervous system included increased heart, pulse, and respiratory rates, sedation, and coma.

Effects resulting from cell membrane disruption included internal hemorrhaging, edema, diarrhea, constriction of the abdominal muscles, and lesions of the stomach and duodenum.

Other short-effects of nightshades:

- Abdominal cramps, gas, diarrhea
- Aphrodisiac symptoms
- Depressed central nervous system
- Depression
- Dizziness
- Eczema, Gout and Allergies
- Flu like illness in higher dosages
- General weakness
- Damage to the gastrointestinal tract as well as to the retina
- Higher concentrations inhibited fibroblast cell growth
- Immune system dysfunctions
- Intestinal Disorders, Overeating
- Kidney inflammation
- Loss of memory, Mental confusion
- Loss of thinking ability
- Loss of night vision
- Premenstrual Syndrome
- Reduced iron, calcium, and oxygen uptake
- Sexual dysfunctions
- Sleepiness
- Vision problems including ocular pressure

Solanine is a cell disruptor (causes the cell to rupture), and attacks the lining of the stomach and intestine.[133] This can be the source for intestinal bleeding, ulcers, and other related issues. Anyone suffering from such disorders should eliminate nightshades plants from their diet in order to identify them as a cause.

Vision: one of the symptoms of nightshades neurotoxins (atropine) is ocular pressure; this causes various vision problems that prevent the eye from focusing properly.[134] The effect is temporary.

## Possible Long Term Effects

- Alzheimer's
- Arthritis
- Birth Defects and Miscarriages
- Cancer
- Congenital spina bifida
- Death (rare, and it is a long term effect)
- Endocrine System Dysfunctions
- Heart Attack
- Osteoporosis
- Parkinson's Disease
- Polio (remittent fever)

---

[133] a-Chaconine [20562-03-2] and a-Solanine [20562-02-1] Review of Toxicological Literature, Prepared for Errol Zeiger, Ph.D., National Institute of Environmental Health Sciences, Submitted by Raymond Tice, Ph.D. ,Integrated Laboratory Systems, February 1998
[134] ANTIDOTES FOR POISONING BY ORGANOPHOSPHORUS PESTICIDES Monograph on Atropine, ANDREW J. HEATH MD PhD

# Arthritis

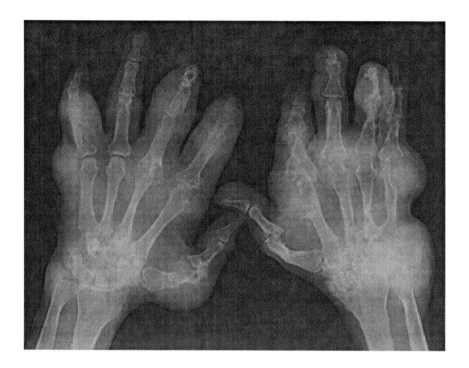

*Severe Arithritis, Photo: Harvard University*

Drs. Childers and Margoles issued a report on the connection between a nightshade diet and arthritis. They used a number of means to identify a positive correlation. The following is a brief summary of that report:

- A survey of people who had arthritis and would eliminate nightshades from their diets to see if their affliction would be reduced.
- A study with rats and nightshades.
- A correlation of arthritis in livestock that have nightshades included as feed.

**The results of the surveys:** by Dr. Childers, Ph.D and M.S. Margo-les, M.D.

- Of the 5000 readers canvassed, 434 returned a questionnaire (8.6%);
- Arthritis had been diagnosed by a physician in 85% of respondents;
- 79% had been treated with drugs, with 80% receiving some degree of temporary relief;
- 52% indicated they were rigidly on the diet, 48% had "slipped" occasionally;
- Rigidly on the diet, 94% had complete or substantial relief from symptoms;
- Of dieters with an occasional "slip" 50% had complete or substantial relief;
- Overall, 68% had complete or substantial relief.

Not everyone is helped by avoiding the family of nightshade plants, but one study showed 75% of those suffering arthritis symptoms experienced relief or remission on the nightshade-free diet.[135]  Response time varied depending on the severity of disease symptoms, joint, tendon and connective tissue damage.  Since solanine is a stable non-water soluble chemical it can take months for your body to rid itself of this toxic substance.

One case I personally was involved with was a woman in her late fifties who had arthritis so bad that she qualified for disability and could no longer perform a simple office job.  After the termination of her work, she became chair bound and could hardly move about the house; simple tasks such as opening jars and cleaning the house were impossible for her.  Her days were spent in pain that often brought her to tears.  Even sleep was difficult.

---

[135] Journal of Neurological and Orthopedic Medical Surgery(1993)12:227-231, *An Apparent Relation of Night-shades(Solanaceae)to Arthritis*, N.F. Childers, Ph.D. and M.S. Margoles, M.D.

She ate potatoes and tomatoes on a daily basis. After eliminating potatoes from her diet, she noticed slight relief. It was not until she removed all nightshades, mainly tomatoes that she dearly loved, did she experience significant relief. She is now active, able to clean the house, and play with the grand children.

This case is typical. It is only with complete elimination of the nightshades can any real results be seen. Most of those affected report that any transgressions can bring back the symptoms vigorously.

### Internet Resources for Arthritis:

- www.thezephyr.com/health/healthmu.htm
- www.noarthritis.com/nightshades.htm
- healthychristianliving.com/rheumatoid_arthritis.htm
- garynull.com/Documents/Arthritis/Prevention_&_Treatment _ of_Osteoarthritis.htm

## Appendicitis

One of the heaviest consumers of potatoes are the not the Irish, but the English. A rare study was done on potatoes and the rate of acute appendicitis in England and Wales. The survey done in 59 different areas, with 49,690 patients, over five years, who had all been discharged from hospitals with acute appendicitis. There was found to be a *statistically significant positive correlation with potato consumption and a negative correlation with non-potato vegetables.*[136]

It may well be that solanine in nightshades are building up in the appendix. Solanine is a cell disruptor, and causes inflammation. Therefore, the reason for the direct correlation of potatoes and appendicitis. If the

---

[136] Vegetable consumption and acute appendicitis in 59 areas in England and Wales. D J Barker, J Morris, and M Nelson, Br Med J (Clin Res Ed). 1986 April 5; 292(6525): 927–930.

study had been done in such a way as to test for all nightshades, rather than just potatoes, the results may have been even more significant.

In the following charts, the minus sign means no correlation and the positive sign a correlation with potatoes, or groups with potatoes included. Also, note the positive correlation with white bread, which is often made with potato water, so it stays soft for days.

TABLE I—*Correlation between food consumption and hospital discharge rates for acute appendicitis in 59 areas in England and Wales*

| | Consumption (g/person/day) | | | Correlation coefficients | |
|---|---|---|---|---|---|
| Food group | Mean | Range | SD | 59 Areas | 20 Exactly matched areas† |
| All vegetables (fresh, frozen, tinned) | 343 | 264-437 | 35·4 | 0·11 | 0·34 |
| Vegetables other than potatoes | 164 | 125-209 | 17·8 | −0·41** | −0·51* |
| Potatoes | 179 | 95-290 | 36·5 | 0·31* | 0·54* |
| Fruit (fresh, frozen, tinned) | 95·1 | 67-125 | 16·4 | −0·27* | −0·22 |
| Bread: | | | | | |
| White | 91·4 | 59-126 | 16·1 | 0·21 | 0·36 |
| Brown/wholemeal | 21·6 | 11·8-34·6 | 4·9 | −0·12 | 0·11 |
| Meat | 157 | 129-184 | 14·6 | −0·06 | −0·24 |
| Fish | 19·4 | 13·3-27·9 | 3·4 | −0·13 | −0·00 |
| Sugar | 46·1 | 35·1-59·0 | 5·5 | 0·30* | 0·23 |

The significant levels of the product moment correlation coefficients (r) for 59 pairs of observations were: >0·26, p<0·05; >0·33, p<0·01; >0·43, p<0·001; and for 20 pairs of observations >0·44, p<0·05; >0·56, p<0·01; >0·68, p<0·001.
*p<0·05. **p<0·01.
†See text.

TABLE II—*Correlation between vegetable consumption and hospital discharge rates for acute appendicitis in 59 areas in England and Wales*

| | Consumption (g/person/day) | | | Correlation coefficients | |
|---|---|---|---|---|---|
| Food group | Mean | Range | SD | 59 Areas | 20 Exactly matched areas† |
| Green vegetables (fresh and frozen) | 58·6 | 26·4-87·8 | 14·8 | −0·33* | −0·52* |
| Cabbage | 16·6 | 9·6-23·6 | 3·8 | −0·34** | −0·36 |
| Cauliflower | 10·4 | 4·4-18·9 | 3·6 | −0·17 | −0·41 |
| Peas | 9·2 | 2·0-15·5 | 3·4 | −0·27* | −0·35 |
| Beans | 8·4 | 0·8-17·6 | 3·9 | −0·20 | −0·32 |
| Brussels sprouts | 7·6 | 2·8-13·8 | 2·2 | −0·48*** | −0·58** |
| Leafy salads | 5·5 | 2·8-10·0 | 1·5 | 0·02 | −0·17 |
| Tomatoes (fresh and processed) | 21·3 | 15·3-30·3 | 3·2 | −0·40** | −0·43 |
| Root vegetables | 23·0 | 12·7-38·2 | 4·9 | −0·13 | −0·09 |
| Onions/leeks | 13·1 | 8·6-19·3 | 2·7 | −0·14 | −0·07 |
| Baked beans | 16·9 | 8·6-24·1 | 2·9 | 0·03 | 0·03 |
| Other (including tinned) | 31·6 | 20·1-42·7 | 5·3 | −0·05 | −0·26 |

*p<0·05. **p<0·01. ***p<0·001.
†See text.

*British Medical Journal: Volume 292, p. 928*[137]

[137] Ibid

TABLE III—*Correlation between consumption of dietary fibre and hospital discharge rates for acute appendicitis in 59 areas in England and Wales*

| Food group | Consumption (g person day) | | | Correlation coefficients | |
|---|---|---|---|---|---|
| | Mean | Range | SD | 59 Areas | 20 Exactly matched areas† |
| All vegetables | 8·8 | 6·7-10·8 | 0·8 | −0·03 | 0·13 |
| Vegetables other than potatoes | 5·5 | 4·3-7·0 | 0·6 | −0·34** | −0·37 |
| Potatoes | 3·3 | 1·4-4·5 | 0·6 | 0·31* | 0·52* |
| Cereals‡ | 8·3 | 7·3-10·7 | 0·6 | 0·07 | 0·26 |
| Bread | 4·2 | 3·6-5·1 | 0·4 | 0·04 | 0·38 |
| Other cereal foods | 4·1 | 3·3-6·9 | 0·5 | 0·05 | 0·11 |
| Total | 19·2 | 16·9-22·3 | 1·3 | −0·02 | 0·28 |

*p<0·05. **p<0·01.
†See text.
‡Calculated according to Paul and Southgate.[13]

*British Medical Journal: Volume 292, p. 929*[138]

# Alzheimer's

(als´himerz, ôls-) , degenerative disease of nerve cells in the cerebral cortex that leads to atrophy of the brain and senile dementia. The disease is characterized by abnormal **accumulation of plaques** and by neurofibrillary tangles (malformed nerve cells), changes in brain tissue first described by Alois Alzheimer in 1906. The plaques result from the release and accumulation of **excessive amounts of beta-amyloid proteins**, normal proteins whose function in the body is not known.

The neurofibrillary tangles prevent transportation of synthesized products within the cell body to organelles and target sites. The plaques and neurofibrillary tangles prevent proper transmission of electrochemical signals necessary for information processing and retrieval. The plaques also suffocate neurons by inhibiting proper blood supplies from reaching them.

Alzheimer's disease usually affects people over age 65, although it can appear in people as young as 40. A condition called mild cognitive impairment, in which a person experiences an inability to form memories for events that occurred a few minutes ago, typically is the first sign of the disease. Although other conditions may cause such impairment, if no identifiable cause is present, mild cognitive impairment leads to Alzheimer's in some 80% of the cases. As the disease progresses, a variety of symptoms

---

[138] Ibid

may become apparent, including loss of memory, confusion, irritability, and restlessness, as well as disorientation and impaired judgment and concentration.

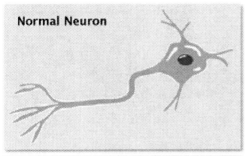

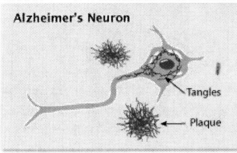

*Alzheimer's Damaged Neuron– The University of Utah, Genetic Science Learning Center*

The cause of Alzheimer's is unknown. Mutations in a gene on chromosome 21, which is also associated with Down's syndrome, and another gene on chromosome 14, have been found in early-onset cases. Late-onset cases, which are the vast majority, may be caused by a combination of genetic and environmental factors. In 1999, scientists discovered an enzyme, named betasecretase, that begins a toxic process in the brain leading to Alzheimer's disease.

There is as of yet no known cure for Alzheimer's. Genetic screening for families with a history of early Alzheimer's is sometimes advised. *"Treatment includes relieving the patient's symptoms and alleviating stress on caregivers through support groups and counseling services. Donepezil (Aricept), rivastigmine (Exelon), and other acetylcholinesterase inhibitors provide temporary improvement for some patients with mild to moderate Alzheimer's."* [139]

The problem with Alzheimer's and nightshades is the sufferers are lacking Acetylcholine (ACh), which is why treatments use Acetylcholinesterase (AChE) inhibitors to increase the amount of free ACh. Nightshades contain AChE inhibitors such as solanine, which may be helpful, but they also contain Atropine which is not beneficial, as it is an ACh blocker. *"Biochemical studies show that choline acetyltransferase, the key enzyme*

---

[139] D. Shenk (2001),Columbia Encyclopedia, Sixth Edition, Alzheimer's Association

*required for the synthesis of acetylcholine, is decreased in the cerebral cortex in Alzheimer's disease."*[140]

*"In vivo administration of **α-chaconine**, (10, 30 and 60 mg/kg) to adult male rats caused a **reduction of brain AchE activity** to 79, 55 and 18% of the control activity for the respective doses."*[141]

Please read the section on Mental Development and "stickiness" of brain-cells. The brain cells of Alzheimer's patients are found to be "sticky"; this issue is one of the top concerns in research. Now, look at the following report.

*Oral administration of 10 mg/kg 3H-a-chaconine to the hamster led to bound residues in lung, liver, kidney, heart, brain, and testes. **Residues in brain and testes were 100% bound** (Alozie et al., 1978b)."*[142]

I may not be the sharpest tack-in-the-box, but if nightshade toxins are binding to brain-cells and Alzheimer's brain-cells have something binding to them, well, it is not much of a jump to do a correlation study for nightshade consumption and Alzheimer's.

Alzheimer's sufferers may benefit from a nightshade free diet in order eliminate Atropine, which may also be an instigator of Alzheimer's, but a connection cannot be determined from published studies.

---

[140] Khosh, Dr. Farhang. *Naturopathic Approach to Alzheimer's Disease*, Townsend Letter for Doctors and Patients, July 1, 2001.

[141] SYDNEY O. ALOZIE, RAGHUBIR P. SHARMA, DATTAJIRAO K. SALUNKHE (1978) *INHIBITION OF RAT CHOLINESTERASE ISOENZYMES IN VITRO AND IN VIVO BY THE POTATO ALKALOID*, α-CHACONINE1,2 Journal of Food Biochemistry 2 (3), 259–276. doi:10.1111/j.1745-4514.1978.tb00621.x

[142] *Inhibition of Human Plasma and Serum Butyrylcholinesterase* (EC 3.1.1.8) by a-Chaconine and a-Solanine; H. N. NIGG, L. E. RAMOS, E. M. GRAHAM, J. STERLING, S. BROWN, AND J. A. CORNELL;University of Florida, I FAS, Citrus Research and Education Center, 700 Experiment Station Road. Lake Alfred. Florida 33850

## Birth Defects and Miscarriages

*"potato glycoalka-loids have embryo toxicity. It could cause the **death of embryos and result in absorbed and dead fetuses.** (3) potato glycoal-kaloids could evidently affect the development of embryos and lead to intrauterine growth retardation (IUGR). **An interesting phenom-ena which just like the clinical manifestation of miscarriage in human being was noticed.** If potato glycoalkaloids were given to the pregnant mice on the 5th or 6th day of gestation intraabdominally, vaginal bleeding and abortion would occur, and this has not been reported yet."* [143]

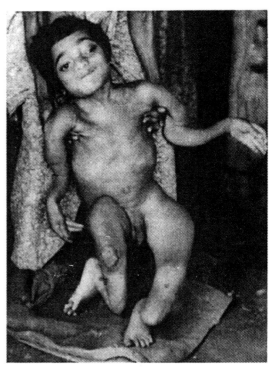

A child with brittle bone disease. (Photo by Philip Kgosana)

Several studies have shown that a-chaconine, and a-solanine, are a cause of birth defects in mammals. The reported abnormalities were as follows: central nervous system abnormalities (e.g., exencephaly[144], cranial bleb, encephalocele[145], and anophthalmia[146]). Some studies found no neural tube defects, but reported a high incidence of other abnormalities, includ-

---

[143]*Teratogenic effect of potato glycoalkaloids;* Zhonghua Fu Chan Ke Za Zhi. 1993 Feb;28(2):73-5, 121-2.Wang XG.Second Teaching Hospital, Bethune University of Medical Sciences, Jilin.

[144] brain is located outside of the skull
[145] neural tube defect
[146] absence of one or both eyes.

ing mild hydronephrosis[147], hydroureter[148], and irregular or fused ribs. Many studies reported miscarriages of the fetus as a direct result from nightshade neurotoxins.

It must be noted that the tropane alkaloids in nightshades reduced calcium uptake by 80%[149], that this may be one of the reasons for the increase in birth defects. The nervous system especially is dependent on a good supply of calcium.

Nightshades have a long history in witchcraft for being used to induce abortions.[150] It is reasonable to suspect that if large amounts of solanine were ingested it may be a cause for a miscarriage or defects of the embryo.

*"The embryo toxicities of two **major potato glycoalkaloids, alpha-chaconine and alpha-solanine,**...Some combinations exhibited strong synergism in the following measures of developmental toxicity: (a) 96-hr LC50, defined as the median concentration **causing 50% embryo lethality**; (b) 96-hr EC50 (malformation), defined as the concentration **causing 50% malformation** of the surviving embryos;"[151]*

*"Daily injections (days 5-12) of 20 and 40 mg/kg of the glycoalkaloid caused **100% fetal and maternal mortality**, respectively. Daily ip injections of 5 mg/kg of solanine into New Zealand White rabbits on days 0-8 of gestation **produced abortion** in one-third of the treated animals, 23% resorptions, but no teratogenesis. Single yolk-sac injections of 5-20 mg/kg of solanine into 20-22 h*

---

[147] distention and dilation of the renal pelvis

[148] Accumulation of urine in and distention of the ureter due to obstructed outflow.

[149] SOLANINE AND CHACONINE:First draft prepared by Dr T. Kuiper-Goodman and Dr P.S.Nawrot Bureau of Chemical Safety Health and Welfare Canada Ottawa, Ontario, Canada

[150] *History of Witchcraft*, By Christina Hole, out of print

[151] *Synergistic interaction of glycoalkaloids alpha-chaconine and alpha-solanine on developmental toxicity in Xenopus embryos.*Rayburn JR, Friedman M, Bantle JA.US Environmental Protection Agency, Environmental Research Laboratory, Gulf Breeze, FL 32561, USA. 1995 Dec;33(12):1013-9.

*incubated white Leghorn eggs* **produced 63-90% mortality** *within 72 h without significant teratogenesis.*[152]

"*Abortion of fetuses occurred in five of 24 pregnant mice on the solanidine and none on the other diets.*"[153]

"*Potatoes, for example, naturally contain the fat soluble neurotoxins solanine and chaconine (49), which can be detected in the bloodstream of all potato eaters. High levels of these potato neurotoxins have been shown to* **cause birth defects** *in rodents (48).*"[154]

Testing oral doses on hamsters: "*A single a-chaconine dose of 200 mg/kg (0.23 mmol/kg) to pregnant Syrian hamsters on day 8 of gestation induced maternal toxicity (incidence ratio not provided) and* **death of all fetuses in 12% of the litters** *(Renwick, 1982). Seven out of eight live litters had at* **least one embryo with malformations** *of the central nervous system (CNS) (i.e., exencephaly and cranial bleb).*"

Testing on rats: "*When solanine was administered at 30 or 40 mg/kg/day (0.03 or 0.05 mmol/kg) to pregnant Holtzman rats through gestation and weaning, an increase in the number of litters in which* **all the pups died was observed** *(Kline et al., 1961). Additionally, the percentage of pups surviving past weaning was reduced from 82.6% in the control group to 31% at both doses.*"[155]

---

[152] *Are potatoes teratogenic for experimental animals?*, Chester A. Swinyard, Shakuntala Chaube, Institute of Rehabilitation Medicine, New York University Medical Center, New York, New York 10016, Teratology, Volume 8, Issue 3 , Pages 349 – 357,Published Online: 10 May 2005

[153] *Effect of feeding solanidine, solasodine and tomatidine to non-pregnant and pregnant mice*,FRIEDMAN Mendel ; HENIKA P. R. ; MACKEY B. E. Food and chemical toxicology (Food chem. toxicol.) ISSN 0278-6915   2003, vol. 41, no1, pp. 61-71

[154] *ENVIRONMENTAL POLLUTION, PESTICIDES, AND THE PREVENTION OF CANCER: MISCONCEPTIONS*\* July 21, 1997 by Bruce N. Ames and Lois Swirsky Gold.

[155] a-Chaconine [20562-03-2] and a-Solanine [20562-02-1] Review of Toxicological Literature, Prepared for Errol Zeiger, Ph.D.,National Institute of Environmental Health Sciences,Submitted by Raymond Tice, Ph.D. ,Integrated Laboratory Systems,February 1998

It seems foolish to risk ingestion of nightshades while pregnant or nursing, considering the possible effects. It is common knowledge that tobacco (a nightshade) is a source of birth defects; it is within reason to suspect all nightshades, since all nightshades contain nicotine even the potato. Tests will never be performed on human embryos, as it would be immoral, thus conclusions will be hard to come by.

One experiment involved monkeys fed a diet of potatoes, *"containing on average 26 mg solanine per 100 g tuber for 25 consecutive days during days following mating. It subsequently apparent that the monkeys were not pregnant."* Nightshades may contribute to miscarriages. 26mg/100g is allowable for human consumption according the World Health Organization. 10mg/100g is the recommended level; however, these recommendations seem misguided since other studies show that nightshade toxin build-up in the system over time.

*"We recommend that a systematic study of the embryotoxicity and tera-togenicity of Solanaceous alkaloids be conducted with the goal of setting a toxicologically based standard for human consumption."* [156]

The U.S. Sheep Experiment Station found that potatoes prevented proper implantation of the embryo.

*"Results indicated that exposure of bovine oocytes[157] to the steroidal glycoal-kaloids during in vitro maturation **inhibited** subsequent pre-implantation embryo development."*[158]

---

[156] *Inhibition of Human Plasma and Serum Butyrylcholinesterase* (EC 3.1.1.8) by a-Chaconine and a-Solanine1 H. N. NIGG,2 L. E. RAMOS, E. M. GRAHAM,3 J. STERLING,3 S. BRWN,3 AND J. A. CORNELL4

[157] Wang, S., Panter, K.E., Gaffield, W., Bunch, T. 2004. *Effects of steroidal glycoalkaloids from potatoes (solanum tuberosum) on in vitro bovine embryo development.* Animal Reproduction Sciences.

[158] *Effects of steroidal glycoalkaloids from potatoes (Solanum tuberosum) on in vitro bovine embryo development.* Wang S, Panter KE, Gaffield W, Evans RC, Bunch TD.US Sheep Experiment Station, USDA-ARS, Dubois, ID 83423, USA. 2005 Feb;85(3-4):243-50.

What this is saying is that nightshades are preventing fertilization of sheep by affecting the egg so it cannot receive the spermatozoa.

## Spina Bifida

Means "split spine" when any one of the 33 vertebrae in the spine does not properly form during the first stages of pregnancy, the nerves in the spine can be left unprotected, thus leading to damage of the central

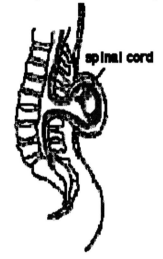

nervous system. Effects include reduced mobility, bladder and bowel problems and even paralysis in areas below the defect.

Simply taking 400 mg of folic acid daily during childbearing years reduces the incidence of spina bifida by 70%.

Spina bifida is one of the most common birth defects: 1-2 cases per 1000 births (world-wide). In the U.S., it is 0.7 per 1000 births. Spina bifida is one type of neural tube defect (NTD) that can also occur in the brain. Most (NTD) occur during the process of neurulation[159], which is the period between day 17 and day 30 after conception,[160] typically before a women is aware of being pregnant. Thus having proper health during childbearing years is very important.

What is the cause of spina bifida? According to the The Irish Association for Spina Bifida & Hydrocephalus, "*The exact cause of Spina Bifida is unknown.*" The occurrence of spina bifida is higher in Ireland than the rest of the world: 4.2 per 1000 births[161]. Guess what is also high in Ireland?

---

[159] Steps of neurulation include the formation of the dorsal nerve cord, and the eventual formation of the central nervous system. The process begins when the notochord induces the formation of the central nervous system (CNS) by signaling the ectoderm germ layer above it to form the thick and flat neural plate. The neural plate folds in upon itself to form the neural tube, which will later differentiate into the spinal cord and the brain, eventually forming the central nervous system.

[160] Lemire RJ (1988). *Neural tube defects.* JAMA 259 (4): 558–62. PMID 3275817.

[161] High-Risk Newborns - Spina Bifida; Robert Wood Johnson University Hospital

Spina Bifida occurs quite often in Wales and in parts of England,[162] both are very high in nightshade consumption. However, when Irish immigrate to the U.S. and marry other Irish the occurrence goes down; currently this is unexplainable, unless you factor in lower consumption of nightshades in the U.S. If it were genetic then the immigration studies would have been able to demonstrate that factor, but the correlation is negative.

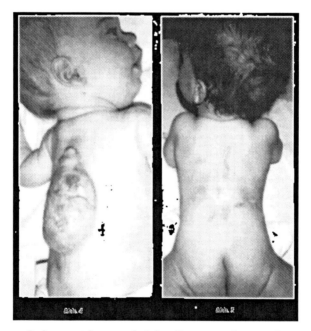

*Infants with spina bifida: Courtesy of www.obgyn.org*

---

[162] *GEOGRAPHICAL NEUROSURGERY*; Congress of Neurological Surgeons: Samuel C. Ohaegbulam, M.B, B.Ch (Cairo), FRCS (Ed), FRCS (Eng), FWACS (W. Africa), FMCS (Nig), FICS

# Rates of neural tube defect by location

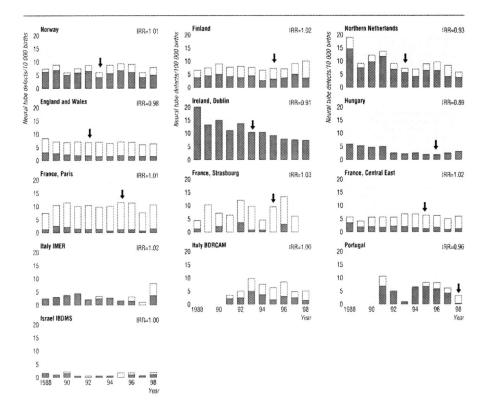

**Chart:** *Rates of neural tube defects (anencephaly and spina bifida) per 10 000 births, 1988-98. Shaded top portion indicates terminated pregnancies. Arrow indicates time of recommendations in each country. IRR=average rate of change from one year to next[163]*

Ireland has the world's highest incidence of Spina bifida, in Belfast, Ireland alone the rate is 144.98/ 10,000[164]and the world's highest rate of potato consumption, 140 kg per capita.[165] That was a positive correlation,

[163] BMJ 2005;330:571 (12 March), doi:10.1136/bmj.38336.664352.82 (published 18 February 2005) *International retrospective cohort study of neural tube defects in relation to folic acid recommendations: are the recommendations working?*
[164] *Malformations* By Pierre J. Vinken
[165] *The Potato In The Food Business Past To Present* by Liam Glennon

go back and look at the of spina bifida for Israel (lowest), if my conclusion is correct then we should see a low consumption of potatoes. The average Israeli eats 34 kilograms of potatoes each year, less than half the 80 kg eaten per capita in the US and Western Europe and the 120 kg eaten by the average resident of Russia and Eastern Europe.[166] Therefore, we see two positive correlations with potatoes and spina bifida. Consumption increases and avoidance decreases the rate of incidence.

Other factors, of course, weigh-in and need to be accounted for, such as consumption of food high in folic acid, etc. A study must be done to see if a direct correlation with nightshade consumption and spina bifida can be found, BEFORE they can be deemed safe for women to eat during childbearing years. At least an education program would be in order.

Some have made the connection to potato fungus and spina bifida, but not to the potato itself. It may well be that two correlations exist.

*"A correlation was identified between the severity of potato late-blight (which causes **increased glycoalkaloid** levels) and the incidences of congenital spina bifida in humans (Renwick, 1972; Renwick et al., 1974). Ireland, with highly suitable weather for blight fungus, has the world's highest incidence of congenital spina bifida (Renwick, 1972)."* [167]

The Centers for Disease Control (CDC) issued a report following an investigation on the incidence of spina bifida, by studying reports from 16 states between 1983 and 1990. *"The results indicated that spina bifida occurred in 4.6 out of 10,000 births. The incidence of the birth defect varied from 3.0 per 10,000 births in Washington to 7.8 per 10,000 births in Arkansas. The CDC plans to recommend that women take folic acid supplements to prevent **neural tube defects** such as spina bifida. The annual medical and*

---

[166] Daniel Kennemer. *Business in brief*, Jerusalem Post, May 2, 2006

[167] a-Chaconine [20562-03-2] and a-Solanine [20562-02-1] Review of Toxicological Literature, Prepared for Errol Zeiger, Ph.D.,National Institute of Environmental Health Sciences,Submitted by Raymond Tice, Ph.D. ,Integrated Laboratory Systems,February 1998

*surgical costs (based on 1985 dollars) for persons with spina bifida exceed $200 million."*[168]

While the above does not relate to nightshades it does show how small changes in diet can dramatically effect the health of the embryo.

Testing on hamsters: *"A high incidence of **neural tube defects** such as interparietal encephalocoele (11-13%) and exencephaly (5-12%) was observed in fetuses, of which the mothers were **exposed to either alpha-chaconine or alpha-solanine**."*[169]

There is a link to nightshades and spina bifida;[170] it may be that prolonged use of nightshades exacerbates any potential for the disease to occur. *"THE HAGUE, Netherlands, Oct 12, 2004 (United Press International via COMTEX) ~ The risk of the congenital birth abnormality of spina bifida can be reduced measurably if the mother simply eats a balanced diet, a report said Tuesday."*[171]

*"Keeler et al. (78) showed that potato sprouts could be teratogens for the central nervous system in the Syrian hamster. We demonstrate here the same teratogenic effect from a British cultivar, Arran Pilot. Most of the activity was traced to the two solanidine triglycosides, alpha-chaconine and, at a higher dose level,*

---

[168] *Spina bifida incidence at birth - United States, 1983-1990*, Morbidity and Mortality Weekly Report, July 10, 1992.

[169] *SOLANINE AND CHACONINE:*First draft prepared by Dr T. Kuiper-Goodman and Dr P.S.Nawrot Bureau of Chemical Safety Health and Welfare Canada Ottawa, Ontario, Canada

[170] *Inhibition of Human Plasma and Serum Butyrylcholinesterase* (EC 3.1.1.8) by a-Chaconine and a-Solanine1 H. N. NIGG,2 L. E. RAMOS, E. M. GRAHAM,3 J. STERLING,3 S. BROWN,3 AND J. A. CORNELL4

[171] *MOTHER'S DIET LINKED TO SPINA BIFIDA*, United Press International, October 12, 2004.

*alpha-solanine. Some possible implications for the study of human **neural-tube defects** are considered"* [172]

Testing on fertile chicken eggs, *"A high incidence of embryo mortality (20-27%) and increased incidence of abnormalities (16-25%) such as cranioschisis, celosoma, cardiac septal defects, rumplessness (absence of tail) and trunklessness (absence of trunk below the wing bud) were observed in treated embryos. The most frequent defect was rumplessness and trunklessness.* [173] The same studies also showed birth defects in hamsters and pigs.

Testing on Rabbits: *"**Incomplete closure of the caudal vertebral column,** [174] and two other fetuses were very small and had shortened appendages. Among 28 fetuses examined in the Alternaria solani blighted potato group, two fetuses exhibited incomplete closure of the caudal vertebral column, one fetus had **a very small brain** (nearly half the normal size) and the cranial cavity was filled with fluid, and two other fetuses were abnormally small in size. All six abnormal fetuses were from different litters. None of the nine fetuses (two litters) from the unblighted potato group were affected."* [175]

In order to determine the toxicity and teratogenicity of potato glycoalkaloids, the effect of potato glycoalkaloids on Kunming pregnant mice were studied. The results showed that: potato glycoalkaloids **have teratogenic effects on embryos of mice.** It could **induce neural tube defects** (NTDs), and may be an important teratogen of NTDs. [176]

.

---

[172] Renwick JH, Claringbold WD, Earthy ME, Few JD, McLean AC *Neural-tube defects produced in Syrian hamsters by potato glycoalkaloids.* [Journal Article]Teratology 1984 Dec; 30(3):371-81.

[173] Ibid

[174] caudal vertebral column, : near the tail of the spinal column.

[175] Ibid

[176] *Teratogenic effect of potato glycoalkaloids;* Zhonghua Fu Chan Ke Za Zhi. 1993 Feb;28(2):73-5, 121-2.Wang XG.Second Teaching Hospital, Bethune University of Medical Sciences, Jilin.

# Cancer

*"a-Chaconine and a-solanine were nominated for testing based on their fre-quent occurrence in high concentrations in commonly ingested foods and the lack of carcinogenicity data for either compound."* [177]

*"To obtain evidence for possible mechanisms of the observed in vivo effects, the four glycoalkaloids (a-chaconine, α-solanine, solasonine and α-tomatine) men-tioned above and the aglycones solanidine and tomatidine were also evaluated in in vitro assays for estrogenic activity.* **Only solanidine** *at 10 µM concentration* **exhibited an increase in the MCF-7 human breast cancer** *cell proliferation assay."* [178]

It is unfortunate there is a lack of carcinogenic studies on the toxins found in nightshades other than the known carcinogenic nicotine. *"No carcinogenicity data were found for either compound."* [179,180] It would stand to reason that such a notorious carcinogenic as nicotine which is found in the nightshade plants would stimulate research on the carcinogenic affects of chaconine and solanine, since the causes of so many cancers in the diges-tive system remain unknown, (throat, stomach, and intestinal) cancers. We know that nicotine is carcinogenic; it makes sense to suspect chaconine and solanine.

Please read the chapter on *Vitamin D and Livestock*, as it has been found that Vitamin D is helpful in preventing cancer and the solanine may interfere with Vitamin D absorption.

---

[177] a-Chaconine [20562-03-2] and a-Solanine [20562-02-1]   Review of Toxicological Literature, Prepared for Errol Zeiger, Ph.D.,National Institute of Environmental Health Sciences,Submitted by Raymond Tice, Ph.D. ,Integrated Laboratory Systems,February 1998

[178] *Effect of feeding solanidine, solasodine and tomatidine to non-pregnant and pregnant mice*,FRIEDMAN Mendel ; HENIKA P. R. ; MACKEY B. E. Food and chemical toxicology (Food chem. toxicol.) ISSN 0278-6915   2003, vol. 41, no1, pp. 61-71

[179] Ibid

[180] *SOLANINE AND CHACONINE*:First draft prepared by Dr T. Kuiper-Goodman and Dr P.S.Nawrot Bureau of Chemical Safety Health and Welfare Canada Ottawa, Ontario, Canada

It is sad that many have come to suspect that the leading cancer organizations are not interested in solving the causes of cancer, but only look towards procuring money for treatment in order to maintain a livelihood.

According to the International Agency for Research in Cancer, *"...80-90 per cent of human cancer is determined environmentally and thus theoretically avoidable."* [181] Environmental causes of cancer include lifestyle factors such as smoking, a diet high in animal products and low in fresh fruit & vegetables, excessive exposure to sunlight, food additives, alcohol, workplace hazards, pollution, electromagnetic radiation, and even certain pharmaceutical drugs and medical procedures.

The investigative reporters Robert Houston and Gary Null concluded that these institutions had become self-perpetuating organizations whose survival depended on the state of no cure. They wrote, *"a solution to cancer would mean the termination of research programs, the obsolescence of skills, the end of dreams of personal glory; triumph over cancer would dry up contributions to self-perpetuating charities and cut off funding from Congress; it would mortally threaten the present clinical establishments by rendering obsolete the expensive surgical, radiological and chemotherapeutic treatments in which so much money, training and equipment is invested.*

*Such fear, however unconscious, may result in resistance and hostility to alternative approaches in proportion as they are therapeutically promising. The new therapy must be disbelieved, denied, discouraged and disallowed at all costs, regardless of actual testing results, and preferably without any testing at all. As we shall see, this pattern has in actuality occurred repeatedly, and almost consistently."* [182]

Research accounted for only 17% of the American Cancer Society's actual expenditures in 2001. Total research expenditures in 2001 were $130,504,000 and this amount increases every year. [183]

President Nixon declared a "war on cancer" in 1971 and launched a $42 billion spending spree. What has 30 years and $42 billion produced? Not much, according to the University of Chicago's Dr. John Bailar. [184]

---

[181] Robert Sharpe, op. cit. 1988, p.47
[182] Hans Ruesch, op.cit. 1992, p.65-66
[183] American Cancer Society, Inc. (2003)
[184] Fox News 2001By Steven Milloy

*"Nightshade Alkaloids cause: depressed central nervous system; kidney inflammation; **cancer**, birth defects; reduced iron uptake"* - Cornell University, toxins.[185]

The following except is from, Environmental Pollution, Pesticides, and the Prevention of Cancer: Misconceptions, *July 21, 1997 by Bruce N. Ames and Lois Swirsky Gold.* Dr. Bruce N. Ames is a Professor of Biochemistry and Molecular Biology and Director of the National Institute of Environmental Health Sciences Center, University of California, Berkeley, CA. He is a member of the National Academy of Sciences and was on their Commission on Life Sciences. He was a member of the National Cancer Advisory Board of the National Cancer Institute (1976-82). One of the major points Dr. Ames makes in his paper is that 99.9% percent of all carcinogens are not from synthetic or man-made origins. The prevention of cancer will come from changes in diet and not from the removal of pesticides. That millions of dollars are being wasted by the EPA and other such organizations, and very little is being spent on the carcinogenic realities of diet. He puts forth some of the known effects of tobacco upon human beings, although it is it not a direct correlation to potatoes, at the present time the studies needed to not exist

*"Smoking contributes to about 35% of U.S. cancer, about one-quarter of heartdisease, and about 400,000 premature deaths per year in the United States (6, 13). Tobacco is a known cause of cancer of the lung, bladder, mouth, pharynx, pancreas, stomach, larynx, esophagus and possibly colon. Tobacco causes even more deaths by diseases other than cancer. Smoke contains a wide variety of mutagens and rodent carcinogens.*

*Smoking is also a severe oxidative stress and causes inflammation in the lung. The oxidants in cigarette smoke-mainly nitrogen oxides-deplete the body's antioxidants. Thus, smokers must ingest two to three times more Vitamin C than non-smokers to achieve the same level in blood, but they rarely do. Inadequate concentration of Vitamin C in plasma is more common among the poor and smokers.*

---

[185] Cornell University *Poisonous Plants Collection*; www.ansci.cornell.edu

Men with inadequate diets or who smoke may damage both their somatic DNA and the DNA of their sperm. When the level of dietary Vitamin C is insufficient to keep seminal fluid Vitamin C at an adequate level, the oxidative lesions in sperm DNA are increased 250% (14-16). Male smokers, compared to non-smokers, have more oxidative lesions in sperm DNA (16) and more chromosomal abnormalities in sperm (17).

Smoking by fathers, therefore, may plausibly increase the risk of birth defects and childhood cancer in offspring (14, 15, 18). A new epidemiological study suggests that the rate of childhood cancers is increased in offspring of male smokers, e.g., acute lymphocytic leukemia, lymphoma, and brain tumors, are increased 3-4 times"

"We (6) estimate that unbalanced diets account for about one-third of cancer risk, in agreement with the earlier estimate of Doll and Peto (3). Low intake of fruits and vegetables is a major risk factor for cancer..."

"Furthermore, epidemiological studies from various parts of the world show that certain natural chemicals in food may be carcinogenic risks to humans; for example, the chewing of betel nuts with tobacco has been correlated with oral cancer."

"Potatoes, for example, naturally contain the fat soluble neurotoxins solanine and chaconine (49), which can be detected in the bloodstream of all potato eaters. High levels of these potato neurotoxins have been shown to cause birth defects in rodents (48)." [186]

Tobacco is a nightshade plant, and contains many of the same neurotoxins as all of the other nightshades including potatoes. Cancer is a major killer, and there are not any studies on the long-term effects of nightshade consumption and cancer. It could very well be that nightshades are a major source of cancer, and we are not paying attention. No one can possibly say that nightshades are the cause of any of the digestive tract cancers, nor is the author suggesting that this is the case, only that it seems quite logical that studies be done in this regard. Since solanine is a cell disruptor, and injuries to cells increase the risk of cancer, it is therefore reasonable to be suspicious of ingestion of nightshade plants.

---

[186] ENVIRONMENTAL POLLUTION, PESTICIDES, AND THE PREVENTION OF CANCER: MISCONCEPTIONS* July 21, 1997 by Bruce N. Ames and Lois Swirsky Gold.

Nicotine is found in all nightshades. Recently, Srikumar Chellappan of the University of South Florida, in Tampa, US, found that nicotine caused a molecule called Raf-1 to bind to a key protein called Rb, which normally suppresses tumors. It maybe the nicotine does not cause cancer but suppresses the body's ability to fight cancer. This was seen when breast cancers were more likely to spread in smoker than in non-smokers.[187] Please see the chapter "Safe Levels," in this book for the amounts of nicotine in nightshades.

It is also quite clear that the institutions that are supposed to "save us" have little interest in doing so, and every interest in having us remain sick, or shall I say profitable. Please do not think that I hope that we adopt a socialist or government controlled medical system. That would only compound the problem. As long as someone other than the status quo stands a chance at making a profit from a cure we will always have hope. With socialized medicine, the small flame of hope will be quickly snuffed out, as it will demand more money to feed the monster of bureaucracy, which never gets smaller, and can create laws to feed itself. With socialized medicine, we will have a system where cures only mean loss of jobs and competition does not exist.

## Chronic Fatigue

One Botanist did research with a Hmong friend from Southeast Asia, where they would cook and eat black nightshade, Solanum nigrum, which is highly toxic, boiling the leaves until they were not bitter. "After months of watching her Hmong friends eat S. nigrum with no apparent ill effects, Duchon finally decided to try some. She gingerly accepted a small portion of this 'vegetable' at lunch. She thought she had weathered her experiment without incident, but as the day wore on, she became unusually fatigued. 'I was so tired I could barely make it home,' says Duchon, who recalls going to bed and sleeping for 14 hours."[188]

---

[187] Journal of Clinical nvestigation (DOI: 10.1172/JCI28164)
[188] Fackelmann, Kathy A.. "Food, drug, or poison? (toxic plants used by tribal cultures as food or medicine) (Cover Story)", Science News, May 15, 1993.

Much of solanine would be leached out into water, which the Hmong tossed out. They would re-boil the nightshade leaves in fresh water until the bitterness would dissipate. By introducing leaves in small amounts to the children, who do not like nightshades, the gradually build up a tolerance to them. Duchon assumed that the Hmong people gradually developed an ability to digest the nightshade toxins, but research shows this conclusion is most likely in error, and that the Hmong build up a "tolerance" for the nightshade.

This tolerance is what is in question, as smokers build up a "tolerance" also, but it is an artificial one, as the body is never able to adapt to the nicotine so as to render it harmless, even if it can break it down over time. It would seem that this "tolerance" is the sort of "tolerance" that comes with addictions rather than health benefits. Medical research on solanine states that the body is not able to process this glycoalkaloid so it simply remains in the body unchanged, until departure.[189]

For years, the author suffered from bouts of fatigue; since removing nightshades, these bouts have disappeared. Many people who suffer from chronic fatigue may wish to eliminate nightshades as a possible cause. One of the common effects from eating nightshades is sleepiness, so if one has a regular diet of nightshades, it is like taking a little sleeping pill at each meal.

*"However, when rabbits were administered greened potatoes for up to 20 days, the animals became dull and inactive after 4 to 6 days. After 10 days, the animals experienced diarrhea, hair loss, and weight loss followed by watering eyes, body rigidity, and dullness. Treatment decreased protein digestibility by 45% starting on day 1 of administration, and one animal died within 10 to 20 days. The estimated glycoalkaloid intake was 49-53 mg/kg/day (0.057-0.062 mmol/kg/day)."* [190]

---

[189] SOLANINE AND CHACONINE: First draft prepared by Dr T. Kuiper-Goodman and Dr P.S. Nawrot Bureau of Chemical Safety Health and Welfare Canada Ottawa, Ontario, Canada

[190] a-Chaconine [20562-03-2] and a-Solanine [20562-02-1] Review of Toxicological Literature, Prepared for Errol Zeiger, Ph.D.,National Institute of Environmental Health Sciences,Submitted by Raymond Tice, Ph.D. ,Integrated Laboratory Systems,February 1998

A simple test you can do to see if you are suffering from nightshade toxins is to avoid them completely for a few days, then eat at least a one or two servings of nightshades during a meal, if you feel sleepy and you did not "stuff yourself" then you should suspect nightshades. I would eat the same meal with potatoes and then without potatoes, every time I included the potatoes it was naptime.

## Depression

It is the author's belief that nightshades cause depressed body functions, and that this organic or bodily depression leads to a type of mental depression that clears up quickly after nightshades are removed from the diet. Since nightshades cause depression of the nervous system and reduced mental function, this bodily depression may exacerbate clinical types of depression.

*"Nightshade Alkaloids cause: depressed central nervous system; kidney inflammation; cancer; birth defects; reduced iron uptake"*–Cornell University, toxins.

In 1999 a nationwide clinical trial was done on Vagus Nerve Stimulation(VNS), by using electrical stimulation therapy which had been used previously to treat epilepsy. The result of the study showed that 40% of treated patients displayed a 50% or greater improvement, using the Hamilton Rating Scale for Depression. According to the same report 18 million Americans suffer from depression; about one million of those have severe treatment-resistant depression.[191] The reason this is important is that Solanine is a depressant to the Vagus nerve, so again it stands to reason that the elimination of nightshades would be an easy and noninvasive test for elimination of depression.

---

[191] *Vagus Nerve Stimulation Successful For Depression*, DALLAS, TX ~ December 16, 1999

## Endocrine System Dysfunctions

Chaconine and solanine have been found to accumulate in the endocrine system. The endocrine system is one of the least understood in the human body; it is suspected that low thyroid condition may be caused by the accumulation of the tropane alkaloids directly in the endocrine glands.

*"Tissues which accumulated a-chaconine and a-solanine included abdominal fat, adrenals, blood, brain, heart, kidney, liver, lungs, muscle, pancreas, spleen, testis, thymus, and thyroid."* [192]

## Eczema, Gout and Allergies

A number of people who have eliminated nightshades from their diet have recovered from eczema and gout. [193] It takes less than a month to see the results after elimination, thus it is extremely easy to test.

According to the American Academy of Allergies, cooked potatoes maybe a source of allergic diseases, *"Allergy to cooked potato responsible for severe allergic disease in infants and young children"* [194]

## Food Poisoning

It is quite likely that a number of food poisoning incidents are a result of nightshades. *"One subject who received the highest dose of TGA (1.25 mg/kg BW) became nauseous and started vomiting about 4 h post-dose, possibly due to local glycoalkaloid toxicity (although the dosis is lower than generally reported in the literature to cause gastro-intestinal disturbances). Most relevant, the clearance of*

---

[192] a-Chaconine [20562-03-2] and a-Solanine [20562-02-1]  Review of Toxicological Literature, Prepared for Errol Zeiger, Ph.D., National Institute of Environmental Health Sciences, Submitted by Raymond Tice, Ph.D. ,Integrated Laboratory Systems, February 1998
[193] allergyadvisor.com/Educational/May03.htm
[194] American Academy of Allergy, *Asthma and Immunology*

*glycoalkaloids usually takes more than 24 h, which implicates that the toxicants may accumulate in case of daily consumption."*[195]

The following case of food poisoning is not necessarily from nightshades; however, it was suspect due to the short period of time for the onset of symptoms to occur 15 minutes. In contrast, a bacterium normally takes 24 hours to cause symptoms. *"Georgia: On March 23, 1998, the Hall County Health Department received a report that students in an elementary school became ill after eating lunch. Health officials obtained food and illness histories from 452 (77%) of the 584 students. A case was defined as nausea, abdominal cramps, vomiting, or diarrhea within 24 hours in a person after eating the school lunch on March 23. Of the 452 students, 155 (34%) had illnesses meeting the case definition.... The median incubation period was approximately 15 minutes (range: 5-25 minutes), and median duration of illness was 4.5 hours (range: 10 minutes-8 hours)... The short incubation periods suggest that a preformed toxin or other short-acting agent was the cause of illness. Possible agents include bacterial toxins (e.g., Staphy-lococcus aureus enterotoxin and Bacillus cereus emetic toxin); mycotoxins (e.g., deoxynivalenol [DON], acetyl-deoxynivalenol, and other tricothecenes), trace metals, nonmetal ions (e.g., fluorine, bromine, and iodine), plant toxins (e.g., alkaloids such as **solanines**, opiates, ipecac, and ergot; lectins such as phytohemagglutinin; and glycosides)..."*[196]

My point is not to say that this case was caused by solanine, it is to show a clear comparison to solanine poisoning and food poisoning, and that solanine poisoning can occur quickly. *"In a recent (1983) poisoning associated with a school lunch programme, 61 of 109 school children and staff in Alberta, Canada, became ill, most within 5 minutes, after eating baked potato."* (Anon, 1984). Solanine poisoning can occur from as little as 5 minutes to as long as 9 hours.

---

[195] *Mensinga TT, Sips AJ, Rompelberg CJ, van Twillert K, Meulenbelt J, van den Top HJ, van Egmond HP Potato glycoalkaloids and adverse effects in humans: an ascending dose study. [Clinical Trial, Journal Article, Randomized Controlled Trial]Regul Toxicol Pharmacol 2005 Feb; 41(1) :66-72.*

[196] *Outbreaks of Gastrointestinal Illness of Unknown Etiology Associated with Eating Burritos ~* United States, October 1997-October 1998, *Morbidity and Mortality Weekly Report,* March 19, 1999.

The symptoms of solanine poisoning are similar to food poisoning. *"A three to four fold elevation of the potato glycoalkloids, solanine and chaconine (a teratogen), caused by a multiplicity of different environmental and physical conditions, has killed more than 30 people and poisoned several thousand. Because the symptoms of poisoning are very similar to bacterial food poisoning, many other thousands of poisonings are thought to go unremarked...5 cattle have died from eating green vine tomatoes containing tomatine. Consumption of 500g of potato at one meal will institute mild poisoning in sensitive people. The (long-term) chronic effects of solanine are unknown..."*[197]

A 70-year-old woman experienced vomiting, diarrhea, and bloody stools after drinking the juice of a potato with a concentration of solanine 15-fold greater than that of a normal potato (Gonmori et al., 1993). The author, at times, has also experienced such effects from drinking tomato juice, and never questioned the juice but thought it was food poisoning or the 24 hr flu. It is likely that children, the elderly and those who are sensitive are suffering from the effects of solanine poisoning rather than other causes, but do not associate the nightshades as the cause.

## Intestinal Disorders

- Irritable Bowel Syndrome

- Crohn's Disease

- Possible cause for misdiagnosis for Celiac Sprue

### Irritable Bowel Syndrome:

---

[197] Anthony Trewavas of the Institute of Cell and Molecular Biology at the University of Edinburgh, UK.(Comment)", Chemistry and Industry, December 20, 2004.

*Glycoalkaloids are naturally occurring toxins in potatoes, which at high levels may induce toxic effects in humans, mainly on the gastrointestinal tract by cell membrane disruption.[198]–Cornell University*

*"...disruption of intestinal barrier integrity in animals with a genetic predisposition to develop IBD, but not in control animals. Similarly, in vivo oral feeding experiments demonstrated that C:S ingestion, at physiologic concentrations, aggravated histologic colonic injury in mice genetically predisposed to developing IBD. CONCLUSION: Concentrations of glycoalkaloids normally available while eating potatoes can adversely affect the mammalian intestine and can aggravate IBD."[199]*

Solanine is a cell disruptor;[200] it causes the small cells in villa of the small intestine to become inflamed and even burst, and quite possibly nightshades are the cause and/or the misdiagnosis of the three intestinal disorders listed above. It has been the author's experience that after eliminating nightshades from my diet, all the cramping in gastrointestinal disorders has disappeared. The ability to digest wheat and milk has returned to normal. Studies have shown that the highest prevalence of IBD is where potato consumption is highest.[201] *"The symptoms of low grade solanine*

---

[198] *Induction of the cholesterol biosynthesis pathway in differentiated Caco-2 cells by the potato glycoalkaloid alpha-chaconine.*Mandimika T, Baykus H, Poortman J, Garza C, Kuiper H, Peijnenburg A.RIKILT – Institute of Food Safety, Wageningen University and Research Centre, P.O. Box 230, 6700 AE Wageningen, The Netherlands; Division of Nutritional Sciences, Cornell University, Ithaca, NY 14853, USA. 2007 Apr 27;

[199].*Potato glycoalkaloids adversely affect intestinal permeability and aggravate inflammatory bowel disease.*Patel B, Schutte R, Sporns P, Doyle J, Jewel L, Fedorak RN. Division of Gastroenterology, Department of Medicine, University of Alberta, Edmonton, Alberta, Canada. 2002 Sep;8(5):340-6

[200] a-Chaconine [20562-03-2] and a-Solanine [20562-02-1] Review of Toxicological Literature, Prepared for Errol Zeiger, Ph.D.,National Institute of Environmental Health Sciences, Submitted by Raymond Tice, Ph.D. ,Integrated Laboratory Systems, February 1998

[201] *Potato glycoalkaloids adversely affect intestinal permeability and aggravate inflammatory bowel disease.*, Patel B, Schutte R, Sporns P, Doyle J, Jewel L, Fedorak RN., Division of Gastroenterology, Department of Medicine, University of Alberta, Edmonton, Alberta, Canada. ,2002 Sep;8(5):340-6.

*poisoning are acute gastrointestinal upset with diarrhea, vomiting and severe abdominal pain."* [202]

*"Disruption of epithelial barrier integrity is important in the initiation and cause of inflammatory bowel disease (IBD). Glycoalkaloids, solanine (S), and chaconine (C) are naturally present in potatoes, can permeabilize cholesterol-containing membranes, and lead to disruption of epithelial barrier integrity. Frying potatoes concentrates glycoalkaloids.* **Interestingly, the prevalence of IBD is highest in countries where fried potatoes consumption is highest**...*disruption of intestinal barrier integrity in animals with a genetic predisposition to develop IBD, but not in control animals"* [203]

*"Potatoes contain antinutritional and potentially toxic compounds including inhibitors of digestive enzymes, hemagglutinins, and glycoalkaloids. Solanum glycoalkaloids are reported to inhibit cholinesterase, disrupt cell membranes, and induce teratogenicity."* [204]

The elimination of nightshades has almost completely eliminated flatulence, and diarrhea. In one case, a man who had suffered chronic diarrhea for most of his life was cured completely by the elimination of nightshades.

In the first human study (2005) of ingestion of mashed potatoes with a control of total glycoalkaloids: *"One subject who received the highest dose of TGA (1.25 mg/kg BW) became nauseous and started vomiting about 4 h post-dose, possibly due to local glycoalkaloid toxicity (although the dosis is lower than generally reported in the literature to cause gastro-intestinal disturbances). Most*

---

[202] *SOLANINE AND CHACONINE* Dr T. Kuiper-Goodman and Dr P.S.Nawrot Bureau of Chemical Safety Health and Welfare Canada Ottawa

[203] *Potato glycoalkaloids adversely affect intestinal permeability and aggravate inflammatory bowel disease.*, Patel B, Schutte R, Sporns P, Doyle J, Jewel L, Fedorak RN., Division of Gastroenterology, Department of Medicine, University of Alberta, Edmonton, Alberta, Canada. ,2002 Sep;8(5):340-6.

[204] *Postharvest changes in glycoalkaloid content of potatoes.* Friedman M, McDonald GM. Western Regional Research Center, U.S. Department of Agriculture, Albany, California 94710, USA.

*relevant, the clearance of glycoalkaloids usually takes more than 24 h, which implicates that the toxicants may accumulate in case of daily consumption.*"[205] Many had previously thought that solanine was not readily absorbable via ingestion, and was rendered harmless by digestion.


## Crohn's Disease:

Crohn's disease affects approximately 400,000 to 600,000 people in North America. [206] Crohn's disease (also known as regional enteritis) is a chronic, episodic, inflammatory condition of the gastrointestinal tract characterized by transmural inflammation (affecting the entire wall of the involved bowel) and skip lesions (areas of inflammation with areas of normal lining in between). Crohn's disease is a type of inflammatory bowel disease (IBD) and can affect any part of the gastrointestinal tract from mouth to anus; as a result, the symptoms of Crohn's disease can vary between affected individuals. The main gastrointestinal symptoms are abdominal pain, diarrhea, which may be bloody, and weight loss. Crohn's disease can also cause complications outside of the gastrointestinal tract such as skin rashes, arthritis, and inflammation of the eye. [207]

The cause of Crohn's disease is unknown. It is not within the scope of this work to thoroughly investigate any connections between Crohn's disease and nightshades; it is simply enough to alert anyone who may be suffering from Crohn's disease that the elimination of nightshade plants from their diet may be beneficial; even if it is not the source of Crohn's disease, it may reduce aggravation. It maybe causing irritation of the walls

---

[205] *Potato glycoalkaloids and adverse effects in humans: an ascending dose study.*Mensinga TT, Sips AJ, Rompelberg CJ, van Twillert K, Meulenbelt J, van den Top HJ, van Egmond HP [Clinical Trial, Journal Article, Randomized Controlled Trial]Regul Toxicol Pharmacol 2005 Feb; 41(1) :66-72.

[206] *The epidemiology and natural history of Crohn's disease in population-based patient cohorts from North America: a systematic review.*Loftus, E. V.; P. Schoenfeld, W. J. Sandborn (January 2002). Alimentary Pharmacology & Therapeutics 16 (1): 51-60. DOI:10.1046/j.1365-2036.2002.01140.x. PMID 11856078.b

[207] Hanauer, Stephen B. (March 1996). "Inflammatory bowel disease". New England Journal of Medicine 334 (13): 841-848. PMID 8596552. Retrieved on 2006-11-10.

of the digestive tract after extended usage by sensitive people, resulting in an ulcer, diverticula, and polyps[208]

Misdiagnosis can occur if the suffer is sensitive to nightshades. High quantities of nightshades in the diet can inflame the bowel even to the point of slight bleeding, thus giving all the signs of Crohn's. By eliminating nightshades, the diagnosis may be nightshade sensitivity, rather than Crohn's. In addition, sufferers may find that elimination of nightshades reduces Crohn's related bowel disorder.

## Celiac Disease:

Dr. Peter Green, M.D. in his book *Celiac Disease, A Hidden Epidemic*, calls celiac disease the most under-diagnosed autoimmune disease. It is an intestinal disease where the lining of the intestines inflame, rupture (at the surface), and even bleed. It is typically thought to be a reaction from the ingestion of wheat and dairy products; Dr. Green is convinced of this.

It is what many thought I had when I was young as I had all of the symptoms, yet did not have the allergies to confirm this. In his book, he recommends potatoes to sufferers, *"Patients who are very ill should eat a few safe and simple foods. This may include rice, baked potatoes..."*[209] This is very typical of the treatment that was suggested when I was ill.

When my diet was wheat and dairy free, the problems persisted. Now that nightshades are eliminated from my diet, all of the symptoms of Celiac disease are gone. It may very well be that when the intestines are irritated from nightshades, that they are no longer able to digest wheat and diary, as they are large proteins. This may be the reason for the misdiagnosis in many people. Nightshade elimination is an easy test for suffers of Celiac disease, and should be a standard first recommendation for elimination of possible causes.

---

[208] Childers N.F., Russo G.M. The Nightshades and health (extensive literature). New Jersey (Somerville) and Florida (3906 NW 31 Pl., Gainesville 32606): Hortic Pub, 1977
[209] Celicac Disease, AHidden Epidemic, Peter Green, M.D., p.173 and p.241

## Liver Toxins

In studies on rats and hamsters, found that solanine will concentrate in the liver. "*Maximum concentrations of radioactivity occurred between 6 to 12 h for all tissues, with the largest concentration in the liver.*"[210]

*Potato solanidine (the only natural pesticide properly investigated) accumulates in the human liver, kidneys and other tissues, (10) it is thought to be released during pregnancy, and it is detectable in human cadavers.*"[211]

The concern with this accumulation is that solanine is a heptotoxic, a toxin to the liver. A copper deficiency in the liver has been seen in livestock.[212]

The following report is stating that the concentrations of solanine in the liver are 100 times that found in the blood, and the levels needed to affect the inhibition of BuChE (Blood Cholinesterase), which hydrolyses butyrylcholine more quickly than ACh, is only 1/100 of the level found in the liver. "*Assuming regular ingestion of potatoes, these blood concentrations might lead to a liver concentration of 106 /xg/g solanine (2.67 X 10"4 M) (Claringbold et al., 1982). Using the ratios above, the a-solanine liver concentration might be 254.4 /xg/ g, and 477 fig/g a-chaconine. These estimated tissue concentrations (2.67 X 10"4 M solanidine, 2.93 X 10~4 M a-solanine, and 5.60 X 10~4 M a-chaconine) are about 1000X those measured in blood serum. These are very crude estimates, but significant inhibition of BuChE was obtained here at 1/ 100 of these numbers (Tables 1, 2, 5). Based on excretion rate and postmortem samples, Claringbold et al. (1982) estimated a biomagnification of 50X with daily intake of potatoes, an estimate refuted by their own postmortem data discussed above.*

[210] SOLANINE AND CHACONINE Dr T. Kuiper-Goodman and Dr P.S.Nawrot Bureau of Chemical Safety Health and Welfare Canada Ottawa

[211] Anthony Trewavas of the Institute of Cell and Molecular Biology at the University of Edinburgh, UK.(Comment), Chemistry and Industry, December 20, 2004.

[212] *Journal of Neurological and Orthopedic Medical Surgery* (1993) 12:227-231 An Apparent Relation of Nightshades (Solanaceae) to Arthritis N.F. Childers, Ph.D., and M.S. Margoles, M.D.

*Unfortunately, relative tissue concentrations of these alkaloids have not been studied in humans.*"[213]

What was of concern for a number of reasons in this study was the irreversible inhibition of BuChE from alkaloids found in these nightshades, meaning that once inhibition has occurred it will not reverse and the body will have to create new BuChE to replace what was lost.

The liver is the great blood processor of the body; it prevents toxins in the digestion tract from entering the blood stream, thus reducing the amount of toxins the blood and body receive. The reason that solanine accumulates in the liver is due to the liver's preventing most of the solanine from entering the bloodstream. By ingesting nightshades on a daily basis, the liver becomes overwhelmed with toxins. It has been the author's experience that a long-standing liver pain has dissipated two years after elimination of nightshades.

## Memory

Since the major neurotoxins interfere with neurotransmission, they will not only prevent proper memory formation, but also installation. As reported earlier in the case of the date rape drug, scopolamine prevents the formation of memories. *Numerous studies in human subjects have demonstrated that drugs which block muscarinic acetylcholine receptors cause impairments in memory for verbal (Ghoneim & Mewaldt, 1975; Peterson, 1977; Crow & Grove-White, 1973) and non-verbal (Flicker, Serby, & Ferris, 1990) stimuli. In monkeys, systemic or local infusions of scopolamine impair encoding of visual stimuli for subsequent recognition (Aigner & Mishkin, 1986; Tang, Mishkin, & Aigner, 1997).*[214]Thus, when you are reading or talking you will be functioning properly but your capacity for memory can be markedly affected. *Scopola-mine impairs the object recognition memory at doses of 0.1, 0.3, and 1 mg/kg in*

---

[213] *Inhibition of Human Plasma and Serum Butyrylcholinesterase* (EC 3.1.1.8) by a-Chaconine and a-Solanine1 H. N. NIGG,2 L. E. RAMOS, E. M. GRAHAM,3 J. STERLING,3 S. BROWN,3 AND J. A. CORNELL4

[214] *Scopolamine Impairs Human Recognition Memory: Data and Modeling* - Seth J. Sherman, Marc W. Howard, Alireza Atri, Michael E. Hasselmo, Chantal E. Stern Department of Psychology Boston University Submitted to Behavioral Neuroscience June 20, 2002

*rats and at doses of 0.3 and 1 mg/kg in mice.*[215]   One of the studies showed how chachine affected the systems, *Symptoms observed at relatively low doses (8 or 10 mg/kg) included sedation, respiratory impairment, and constriction of abdominal muscles.*[216]

Earlier we talked about how nightshade alkaloids remained bound in the body.  Some of the tests shown were only tests of the overall retention of alkaloids; when specific testing is done on animals the results are stunning:

*"Unfortunately, relative tissue concentrations of these alkaloids have not been studied in humans.  The excretion of a-chaconine and a-solanine in the rat is different from that in man (Norred et al., 1976); hamster excretion of a-solanine is comparable to human excretion of this compound (Alozie et al., 1979; Claringbold et al., 1980; Groen et al., 1993).  Oral administration of 10 mg/kg 3H-a-chaconine to the hamster led to bound residues in lung, liver, kidney, heart, brain, and testes.  **Residues in brain and testes were 100% bound** (Alozie et al., 1978b)."*[217]

An interesting case study involved a 17-year-old boy who was admitted to the emergency room after eating Jimson Weed seeds.  It took 36 hours to recover enough to recall what happened.

*"Following discharge from the hospital, the patient continued to be unable to remember events that occurred after ingestion of the seeds but was able to recall clearly the afternoon of the day he took the seeds.  He had been watching television with friends.  They were eating snacks and he was offered some seeds that were*

---

[215] The object recognition task in rats and mice: A simple and rapid model in safety pharmacology to detect amnesic properties of a new chemical entity; V. Bertaina-Anglade, E. Enjuanesa, D. Morillona and C. Dr. Journal of Pharmacological and Toxicological Methods; Volume 54, Issue 2, September-October 2006, Pages 99-105

[216] *EFFECTS OF a-CHACONINE ON BRAIN BIOGENIC AMINES, ELECTROENCEPHALOGRAM, CARDIAC RATES AND RESPIRATORY RESPONSE IN RATS;* CHARLES N. ALDOUS, R. P. SHARMA, D. K. SALUNKHE Toxicology Program Department of Animal, Dairy and Veterinary Sciences Utah State University Logan, Utah 84322

[217] *Inhibition of Human Plasma and Serum Butyrylcholinesterase (EC 3.1.1.8) by a-Chaconine and a-Solanine;* H. N. NIGG, L. E. RAMOS, E. M. GRAHAM, J. STERLING, S. BROWN, AND J. A. CORNELL;University of Florida, I FAS, Citrus Research and Education Center, 700 Experiment Station Road. Lake Alfred. Florida 33850

*identified as jimson weed seeds.  He assumed they were similar to pumpkin or sunflower seeds.*"

While it is true most of us never need Jimson Weed seed, it does establish that memory blocking effects of nightshade plants.  It has been shown elsewhere that even when nightshade overdose symptoms are not visible the body and mind are still being affected.  When we want to maintain proper mental health, and avoid Alzheimer's and senility, we should avoid nightshades.  The fact of nightshade toxins bonding with the brain should prevent one from thinking that these toxins are safe.

## Mental Development and Schizophrenia

In a recent study published in Environmental Health Perspectives, October 2005, it was found that organophosphates affect not only the proper functioning of the nervous system, but can directly attack devolving brain systems.  They tested Diaxinon, an organophosphate, which has similarities to solanine as a pesticide.  They work in the same way attacking the nervous system.  My concern is whether the pesticide actions of solanine have similar effects on the mental development of embryos in the womb.

We know that mental formation of rats and mice are affected: "*neurotoxicants that directly target developing monoamine terminals tend to produce sprouting further along the axon, thus producing the corresponding increment in the forebrain, which contains the terminal zone.*" [218]   See the section on Birth Defects in this chapter.  These agents are affecting the ability of the nervous system to send signals in the developing child.  "*The two agents also differed in their effects on the 5HT transporter.  Diazinon evoked a decrease in the brainstem and an increase in the forebrain, again similar to that seen for chlorpyrifos ; this pattern is typical of damage of nerve terminals and reactive sprouting...One of the*

---

[218] *Organophosphate Insecticides Target the Serotonergic System in Developing Rat Brain Regions: Disparate Effects of Diazinon and Parathion at Doses Spanning the Threshold for Cholinesterase Inhibition*, Theodore A. Slotkin,1,2 Charlotte A. Tate,1 Ian T. Ryde,1 Edward D. Levin,1,2 and Frederic J. Seidler1;1Department of Pharmacology and Cancer Biology, and 2Department of Psychiatry and Behavioral Sciences, Duke University Medical Center,

*major concerns for human health is the propensity of these agents to produce developmental neurotoxicity,* **even when exposures are too low to elicit signs of systemic intoxication** *(Landrigan 2001,et al)... multiple mechanisms target neural cell replication and differentiation, axonogenesis and synaptogenesis, and the development and programming of synaptic activity, culminating in behavioral deficits (Barone et al. 2000; Casida and Quistad 2004; Gupta 2004; Pope 1999; Qiao et al. 2002, 2003; Yanai et al. 2002)* [219]

Schizophrenia is now being considered a birth defect, meaning that when the brain cells are examined, they do not line up normally. "*A significant difference in cell disorganization was found between schizophrenic and control subjects.*"[220] It is believed that "something" is acting upon the mechanism that coordinates this formation process. It is far too complicated to discuss here, but what is seen is that when the cells travel down a guide wire that directs proper neuron placement of new cells, the cells seem to become "stuck" on the wire, thus misalignment occurs.

"*A variety of maternal infections have been implicated in the risk for schizophrenia, and it has been proposed that inflammatory responses to infection, especially responses that involve cytokines generated by the mother, placenta, or fetus, represent a common mechanism (29). Inflammatory cytokines generated in response to maternal infection can have a* **neurotoxic effect on developing neurons** *(30, 31), and cytokines regulate neurodevelopmental processes implicated in schizophrenia, such as programmed cell death and synapse development.*"[221]

---

[219] *Organophosphate Insecticides Target the Serotonergic System in Developing Rat Brain Regions: Disparate Effects of Diazinon and Parathion at Doses Spanning the Threshold for Cholinesterase Inhibition,* Theodore A. Slotkin,1,2 Charlotte A. Tate,1 Ian T. Ryde,1 Edward D. Levin,1,2 and Frederic J. Seidler1;1Department of Pharmacology and Cancer Biology, and 2Department of Psychiatry and Behavioral Sciences, Duke University Medical Center,

[220] *Hippocampal pyramidal cell disarray in schizophrenia as a bilateral phenomenon,* A.J. Conrad, T. Abebe, R. Austion, S. Forsythe and A. B. Scheibel, Department of Anatomy and Cell Biology, UCLA Medical Center 90024.

[221] *Recent Advances in the Neurobiology of Schizophrenia;* Seiya Miyamoto1, Anthony S. LaMantia2, Gary E. Duncan3, Patrick Sullivan3, John H. Gilmore3 and Jeffrey A. Lieberman3,1 St. Marianna University School of Medicine, Kawasaki 216-8511, Japan and 2 Department of Cell Molecular Physiology 3 Mental Health Neuroscience Clinical Research Center, School of Medicine University of North Carolina, Chapel Hill, NC 27599

Now combine that "neurotoxic effect" with the other tests that show the neurotoxic effects such as the following:

*"The results showed that: (1) potato glycoalkaloids have teratogenic effects on embryos of mice. It could induce neural tube defects (NTDs), and may be an important teratogen of NTDs. (2) potato glycoalkaloids have embryo toxicity."*[222]

It is not a huge leap to say that if schizophrenia is caused by a neurotoxic effect and that nightshades are neurotoxic to developing embryos, that nightshade consumption promotes schizophrenia. It may also promote other mental illnesses that were heretofore unknown. It is evidence from twin and adoption studies that strongly implicates genetic factors in schizophrenia, but those studies which rule out environment, in the nature vs. nurture debate, do not account for the mother's consumption of nightshades before and during pregnancy.

The entire reason that influenza was mentioned in the earlier study is because influenza has a tendency to cause "stickiness" within cells, and researchers have found schizophrenic cells to be "sticky." These same researchers are now looking for causes of that "stickiness." Because some of the nightshade neurotoxins have 100% bonding with brain cells, they become likely suspects.

Furthermore, since new cells are created every twenty days, in the correct conditions, avoiding nightshades may well indeed reduce the effects of schizophrenia, as proper cell alignment will start to occur. It is important to have a healthy diet, plenty of rest and low stress for cell renewal to occur.

With the preceding in mind, it should also follow that a lack of nightshades in the diet swuld increase proper mental growth in non-sufferers as well, leading to increased memory, awareness, intelligence, and other factors of mental well-being. *Cells aged between about 4 and 6 weeks were easier to activate, and displayed a greater degree of activation than younger or*

---

[222] *Tetatogenic effect of potato glycoalkaloids*; Zhonghua Fu Chan,Ke Za Zhi. 1993 Feb; 28(2):73-5, 12 1-2. Wang XG. Second Teaching Hospital, Bethune University of Medical Sciences, Jilin

*older cells, suggesting there is a critical window in their development during which the cells are more "plastic."*[223]

I personally think that if research is done, we will see the following results. Schizophrenia is partly due to misaligned neurons, and that nightshades are disruptive to neuron-formation in development, thus there should be a positive correlation between mental disorders and the use of nightshades by mothers.

We should also see that continued use of nightshades harms proper mental operations and growth even into adulthood.

## Migraine Headaches

It was once thought that migraines were due to problems with blood vessels. Brain imaging (neuroimaging) discovered that during migraines neurological activity is depressed over an area of the cortex[224]. This new phenomenon, called *cortical spreading depression*, is thought to be the cause of migraines.[225] This results in a release of inflammatory mediators that trigger irritation of the cranial nerve roots, mainly the trigeminal nerve[226].

Neuroimaging has shown that a spreading depolarization starts about 24 hours before the migraine occurs. The neurotoxins in nightshades are an obvious suspect. Although I have not been able to do a true experiment, two cases of severe migraine sufferers that eliminated nightshades completely from their diet, have experienced 100% relief. While this may not be true in every case, to eliminate nightshades as a cause of

---

[223] *Adult-formed brain cells important for memory;* 17:27 23 May 2007, NewScientist.com news service, Linda Geddes

[224] Cohen AS, Goadsby PJ (2005). *Functional neuroimaging of primary headache disorders.* Curr Pain Headache Rep 45 (9): 141-146.

[225] Lauritzen M. (1994). *Pathophysiology of the migraine aura. The spreading depression theory;.* Brain 117 (1): 199-210. PMID 7908596.

[226] The trigeminal nerve (the fifth cranial nerve, also called the fifth nerve or simply V) is responsible for sensation in the face. It is similar to the spinal nerves C2-S5 that are responsible for sensation in the rest of the body. Sensory information from the face and body is processed by parallel pathways in the central nervous system.

such a debilitating disorder is beyond question. Since we know that atropine found in nightshades is a depressant of the central nervous system, and that migraines are symptomatic of a depressed nervous system, one does not have to consider the logic for very long.

The following is proof that chaconine, a neurotoxin found in nightshades, does indeed suppress brain function, at least in rats.

*"In vivo administration of $\alpha$-chaconine, (10, 30 and 60 mg/kg) to adult male rats caused a reduction of brain AchE activity to 79, 55 and 18% of the control activity for the respective doses."*[227]

Since there is direct evidence of migraines with suppressed brain function and nightshades suppress brain function, then it follows that nightshades can be a direct cause of migraines.

If nightshades are the cause of migraines, then complete elimination will stop attacks nearly immediately, with the exception of people who have high levels of nightshade neurotoxins in the bloodstream or accumulated elsewhere in the body. Nevertheless, in time complete relief should be found.

It is the author's belief that nightshades are the direct cause of migraines, as the evidence for this point is overwhelming.

Here is a letter from one of the readers:

Dear Michael Fowler,

Thank you so much for your information on the effect of nightshades on migraine headaches. I have been a migraine sufferer since I was a teenager. As you know, there are various theories as to the causes and cures for migraines.

They range from stress, barometric pressure, hormones to various foods considered to be vasal constrictors.[228] I myself have tried a variety of medications for this disorder and found little to no help. I am a psychotherapist in private practice and treat people who are also migraine sufferers. There is little to offer in the way of real relief.

---

[227] SYDNEY O. ALOZIE, RAGHUBIR P. SHARMA, DATTAJIRAO K. SALUNKHE (1978) *INHIBITION OF RAT CHOLINESTERASE ISOENZYMES IN VITRO AND IN VIVO BY THE POTATO ALKALOID, $\alpha$-CHACONINE*1,2 Journal of Food Biochemistry 2 (3), 259-276. doi:10.1111/j.1745-4514.1978.tb00621.x

[228] Vasal constrictors: reducing blood flow in the relevant blood vessels.

When I read your information on the effect of nightshades, I started to wonder if that might be a real trigger. I would often get a migraine on Fridays and I was wondering what the correlation might be. I realized that I often ate vegetable soup with tomatoes in it. The next day I would have a migraine! I also checked the gluten free flour that I use and discovered that it contains potato flour! Those are the only nightshades that I am aware of in my diet.

So I decided to keep a journal of my migraines for a few months. The following is what I discovered.

| | |
|---|---|
| 10-23-06 | Chocolate |
| 11-07-06 | Tomato Soup |
| 11-10-06 | White Chocolate |
| 11-23-06 | Tomato Soup and Stress |
| 12-26-06 | Potatoes |
| 1-5-07 | Tomato Soup |
| 1-21-07 | Tomato Soup |
| 1-26-07 | Tomato Soup |
| 2-29-07 | Tomato Soup |
| 3-9-07 | Tomato Soup |

After reading your material, I stopped eating anything that contained nightshades and I have not had another migraine since! I honestly do not have words for the relief. I know that this information and careful analysis of dietary habits will help millions of migraine sufferers like myself. Thank you again for your dedication to this research.

Yours Truly,

Katherine T.


## Overeating and Malnourishment

All nightshades contain atropine, which is an anesthesia. In some cases, the anesthetic effect of atropine in nightshades can disturb the body's signals from stomach to the brain, which allows a person to know when they are full. The anesthetic effects also seem to inhibit the body's natural enzyme production that aid in digestion. These two problems cause a chain reaction: eating more than one should, not processing the food properly, and not digesting the proper nutrients. Since nightshades can also be responsible for diarrhea, which further inhibits absorption of nutrients, the person then enters a vicious cycle of overeating as they find themselves deprived of the vital nutrients.

*"However, when rabbits were administered greened potatoes for up to 20 days, the animals became dull and inactive after 4 to 6 days. After 10 days, the animals experienced diarrhea, hair loss, and weight loss followed by watering eyes, body rigidity, and dullness.* **Treatment decreased protein digestibility by 45% starting on <u>day one</u> of administration,** *and one animal died within 10 to 20 days. The estimated glycoalkaloid intake was 49-53 mg/kg/day (0.057-0.062 mmol/kg/day)."* [229]

## Parkinson's Disease

Afflicts approximately 1 million to 1.5 million people in the U.S., most of whom are 60 years old or older. The disorder is seen in people of all ethnic groups and among men and women in equal numbers. There is no known cause and no cure, just treatments to help control the symptoms of trembling arms and legs, trouble speaking, and difficulty coordinating movement. Parkinson's disease occurs when neurons degenerate (lose the ability to function normally) in a part of the brain called the substantia nigra. Many of these neurons that degenerate contain the neurotransmitter called dopamine. As these neurons degenerate, dopamine levels fall, and the balance between dopamine and other neurotransmitters, such as acetylcholine, is thrown off. This neurotransmitter imbalance affects the

---

[229] a-Chaconine [20562-03-2] and a-Solanine [20562-02-1] Review of Toxicological Literature, Prepared for Errol Zeiger, Ph.D.,National Institute of Environmental Health Sciences,Submitted by Raymond Tice, Ph.D. ,Integrated Laboratory Systems,February 1998

way muscles work and leads to movement problems. [230] Nightshade neuro-toxins will only exacerbate these conditions.

## Polio (remittent fever)

"*SOLANIN, a poison that is formed in frozen potatoes was found to be the cause of an epidemic in Ireland. The disease had <u>polio-like</u> reactions but was called remittent fever. Old, sprouting potatoes and those that have been exposed to the sun in the growing period until the skin was green were also found to contain this toxic substance.*" –Eleanor McBean, The Hidden Dangers of Polio Vaccine"

Solanine is always in potatoes and it is not formed only when frozen. Levels of solanine increase in cold weather. Old, green, sun ripened, bruised potatoes have very high solanine content. In addition, the Irish Lumper potato is very high in solanine to begin with.

One further problem is that not all farmers are informed of this problem, nor is the public. Cold weather harvesting warnings are not mentioned in agriculture web sites, nor is there a regulation against harvesting after cold weather.

## Osteoporosis, Rickets, and Vitamin D

More than 50 million Americans have arthritis and more than 60% of women over age 65 have osteoporosis. Tropane alkaloids found in nightshade plants have been found to reduce calcium uptake by 80%. Other studies have suggested that these alkaloids remove calcium from the body, whether it be the bones, or from the calcium in the nerve linings, which leads to osteoporosis or nerve damage. Once these tropane alkaloids have bonded with calcium they collect in the soft tissues of the joints, which stimulates inflammation and leads to arthritis. [231] "*Solanine (100 µM*

---

[230] The Journal of the American Medical Association, March 24, 2000

[231] Journal of Neurological and Orthopedic Medical Surgery (1993) 12:227-231

*at pH 7.4) caused a 90% inhibition of active calcium transport in rat duodenum. The inhibition of active calcium transport was accompanied by a 40% decrease in oxygen consumption"* [232] Another connection seems to be Vitamin D interference, covered later.

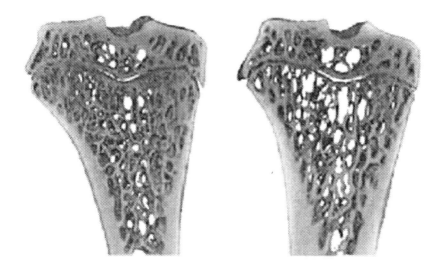

*Image: Osteoporosis showing loss of bone volume, Rat. Normal is on the left, and the affected is on the right (Oregon State University)*

---

[232] SOLANINE AND CHACONINE Dr T. Kuiper-Goodman and Dr P.S.Nawrot Bureau of Chemical Safety Health and Welfare Canada Ottawa

## Vitamin D3

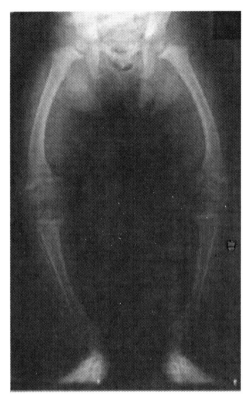

*Image: Two-year child with Rickets*

Vitamin D₃ (*Vitamin D or activated 7-dehydrocholesterol cholecalciferol*)[233] a vitamin that is needed for calcium and phosphorus metabolism. It is found in most fish-liver oils, butter, brain, and egg yolk and is formed in the skin, fur, and feathers of animals and birds exposed to sunlight or ultraviolet rays. Vitamin D₃ is needed for healthy bones and teeth. Rickets is due to a lack of Vitamin D, which results in soft bones in children. This is why milk is fortified with Vitamin D. A lack of Vitamin D as the source of Rickets was discovered by Edward Maloney in 1918-1920, as well as other medical problems.

Rickets was a major problem in the U.S. up until the 1930's when Vitamin D was added to milk.[234] Vitamin D plays an important role in the maintenance of several organ systems. Vitamin D regulates the calcium and phosphorus levels in the blood by promoting their absorption from food in the intestines, and by promoting re-absorption of calcium in the kidneys. It promotes bone formation and mineralization and is essential in the devel-

[233] *vitamin D3*, The Mosby Medical Encyclopedia, October 1, 1996.
[234] Holick MF (2004). *Sunlight and vitamin D for bone health and prevention of autoimmune diseases, cancers, and cardiovascular disease.* American Journal of Clinical Nutrition,80 (6): 1678S-1688S.

opment of an intact and strong skeleton. It inhibits parathyroid hormone secretion from the parathyroid gland. Vitamin D affects the immune system by promoting immunosuppression and anti-tumor activity. Vitamin D stored in the human body as calcidiol (25-hydroxy-vitamin D) has a large volume of distribution and a long half-life (about 20 to 29 days). Vitamin D deficiency tends to increase the risk of infections, such as influenza and tuberculosis. In a 1997 study, Ethiopian children with rickets were 13 times more likely to get pneumonia than children without rickets.[235]

In 2005, scientists released a study which demonstrated a beneficial correlation between Vitamin D intake and prevention of cancer. Drawing from a meta-analysis of 63 published reports, the authors showed that intake of an additional 1,000 international units (IU) (or 25 micrograms) of vitamin D daily reduced an individual's colon cancer risk by 50%, and breast and ovarian cancer risks by 30%. Research has also shown a beneficial effect of high levels of calcitriol on patients with advanced prostate cancer.[236,237]

Vitamin D is also used in the immune system. The hormonally active form of vitamin D mediates immunological effects by binding to nuclear vitamin D receptors (VDR) which are present in most immune cell types, including both innate and adaptive immune cells. The VDR is expressed constitutively in monocytes and in activated macrophages, dendritic cells, NK cells, T and B cells. In line with this observation, activation of the VDR has potent anti-proliferative, pro-differentiative, and immunomodulatory functions including both immune-enhancing and immunosuppressive effects[238]

The following studies seem to show that solanine can have a Vitamin $D_3$ like behavior that interferes with bone growth. In other words,

---

[235] *Case-control study of the role of nutritional rickets in the risk of developing pneumonia in Ethiopian children* Lancet. 1997 Jun 21;349(9068):1801-4..,Muhe L, Lulseged S, Mason KE, Simoes EA., Department of Pediatrics and Child Health, Faculty of Medicine, Addis Ababa University, Ethiopia.

[236] Beer T, Myrthue A (2006). *Calcitriol in the treatment of prostate cancer.* Anticancer Res 26 (4A): 2647-51. PMID 16886675

[237] *Vitamin D 'aids lung cancer ops',* BBC News, 22 April 2005. Retrieved on 2006-03-23.

[238] Nagpal, Sunil, Songqing Naand and Radhakrishnan Rathnachalam (2005) *Noncalcemic Actions of Vitamin D Receptor Ligands,* Endocrine Reviews 26 (5): 662-687.

solanine is being used by the body **as if** it were Vitamin D. The effects of solanine may be widespread, if it indeed is an agent of interference for Vitamin D. The evidence that it interferes with bone growth suggests this.

### Studies on Rats:

Stankiewicz and Evans at Rutgers University performed two experiments to determine if the white potato (Solanum tuberosum), as in the case of Solanum malacoxylon, can naturally produce vitamin D3 and cause pathology in rats as in livestock.

**Trial One:** The rats were fed whole dried potato, some containing vitamin D3 and some not. The diets varied in the amount of potato fed to the different groups of rats. Rats would receive, 0, 5, 15, 25, or 35% whole dried potato in their diet.

**Trial Two:** The levels of dried potato peel were increased which contained increased amounts of solanine, compared to the potato flesh. Rats were either fed 0 or 50% potato in their diet.

**The Results of the Trials:** *"low levels of potato increased bone mineralization due to a hypothesized increase in the intestinal absorption of Ca, P, and Mg. Conversely, a high intake of potato resulted in (1) decreased bone mineral content, (2) soft tissue mineralization, and (3) a decrease in body weight gain. The overall effect indicated the potato does have vitamin D-like activity."*[239]

The above trial demonstrates that nightshades do contain many minerals and vitamins, but increased use leads to decreased bone mineralization (Osteoporosis), the depositing of minerals in the soft tissues, which can be the cause of arthritis, and disturbance of intestinal function, which leads to loss of weight. *"Osteoarthritis appears to be a result of long-term consumption and/or use of the Solanaceae which contain naturally the active metabolite, vitamin D3, which in excess causes crippling and early disability (as seen*

---

[239] Journal of Neurological and Orthopedic Medical Surgery (1993) 12:227-231

*in livestock). Rigid omission of Solanaceae, with other minor diet adjustments, has resulted in positive to marked improvement in arthritis and general health."* [240]

### Livestock:

It has long been known that when livestock feed on nightshade plants certain ill effects will follow: arteriosclerosis, hypercalcemia, parathyroid atrophy, C cell hyperplasia, osteoporosis, osteonecrosis, soft tissue calcinosis, and early death. Most livestock will avoid nightshades that are found in pasture.

Based on livestock research, vitamin D3 found naturally in the nightshades is now being used as a highly effective rat poison[241] at 0.075%. *"the ability of the Solanaceae (those species analyzed) to develop naturally the very active metabolite of vitamin D3 (1a25 dihydroxycholecalciferol) that results in calcinosis of soft tissues, ligaments, and tendons, mineralization in walls of major arteries and veins, and osteopetrosis and related pathology in livestock."* [242]

When these inhibitors accumulate in the body, alone or with other cholinesterase inhibitors such as caffeine or food impurities containing systemic cholinesterase inhibiting pesticides, the result may be a paralytic-like muscle spasm, aches, pains, tenderness, inflammation, and stiff body movements. These symptoms may dissipate in a few hours or days if ingestion is stopped; people vary in sensitivity.

---

[240] Journal of Neurological and Orthopedic Medical Surgery (1993) 12:227-231 An Apparent Relation of Nightshades (Solanaceae) to Arthritis N.F. Childers, Ph.D., and M.S. Margoles, M.D.
[241] SYDNEY O. ALOZIE, RAGHUBIR P. SHARMA, DATTAJIRAO K. SALUNKHE (1978) INHIBITION OF RAT CHOLINESTERASE ISOENZYMES IN VITRO AND IN VIVO BY THE POTATO ALKALOID, α-CHACONINE1,2 Journal of Food Biochemistry 2 (3), 259-276. doi:10.1111/j.1745-4514.1978.tb00621.x
[242] Journal of Neurological and Orthopedic Medical Surgery (1993) 12:227-231 An Apparent Relation of Nightshades (Solanaceae) to Arthritis N.F. Childers, Ph.D., and M.S. Margoles, M.D.

*Hence, in some places, the plant is harmless while it can be toxic in others. Nevertheless, the commonest source of solanine poisoning in farm animals has been with potato tubers, and most cases of solanine poisoning have occurred in European countries.*

*Solanine is poorly absorbed from the gastrointestinal tract, has a rapid fecal and urinary excretion, and hydrolyses to the less toxic and poorly absorbed solanidine. Animal species differ considerably in reaction to solanine toxicity and little is known about the chronic (long-term) toxicity of solanine.[243]*

For access to the full report by Childers and Margoles, please see:

- www.noarthritis.com
- Journal of Neurological and Orthopedic Medical Surgery (1993) 12:227-231 An Apparent Relation of Nightshades (Solanaceae) to Arthritis, N.F. Childers, Ph.D., and M.S. Margoles, M.D.
- Arthritis Nightshades Research Foundation, 177 San Ramon Drive, San Jose, CA 95111-3615, USA.

## Sources of Vitamin D

In many countries, foods such as milk, yoghurt, margarine, oil spreads, breakfast cereal, pastries, and bread are fortified with vitamin D2 and/or vitamin D3, to minimize the risk of vitamin D deficiency. In the United States and Canada, for example, fortified milk typically provides 100 IU per glass, or one quarter of the estimated adequate intake for adults over the age of 50. Fortified foods represent the major dietary sources of vitamin D, as very few foods naturally contain significant amounts of vitamin D. Natural sources of vitamin D include:

- Fish liver oils, such as cod liver oil, 1 Tbs. (15 mL) provides 1,360 IU
- Salmon, cooked, 3.5 oz provides 360 IU
- Mackerel, cooked, 3.5 oz, 345 IU
- Sardines, canned in oil, drained, 1.75 oz, 250 IU

---

[243] *How toxic is Eastern Black Nightshade?*, Weed Science, Univeristy of Wisconsin, Comfort Ateh and Jerry Doll,

- Tuna, canned in oil, 3 oz, 200 IU
- Eel, cooked, 3.5 oz, 200 IU
- One whole egg, 20 IU
- Shiitake mushrooms, one of a few natural sources of vegan and kosher vitamin D (in the form of ergosterol vitamin D2)

## Wheat and Dairy Allergies

Many people who have what seems to be an allergy to wheat and dairy may find that it is the diet of nightshades that inflames the intestines, which in turn prevents proper digestion of these two items. Wheat are dairy are very hard to digest and when the digestive ability is inhibited, these probably start to rot in the gut, causing various types of distress. It was the authors and other experience that once nightshades were removed from the diet that the ability to digest wheat and dairy returned to normal and the production of intestinal gas was nearly completely eliminated. If a person suffers from wheat and dairy allergy it is important to understand if it is a "true" allergy meaning that consumption results in a histamine reaction, or a "false" allergy which is just an inability to properly digest wheat and diary. It is the latter, after a couple of weeks of strict nightshade free dieting, a person can "test" one of the food, by taking a small sample and then waiting 48 hours to see if any symptoms result.

When testing may sure you are in a safe place where you can lay down if need be and have friends around. If symptoms do not occur, then slowly increase the amount until a full serving is had. If you find that wheat gives you no symptoms, you can then try milk. But, first stop eating wheat for 72 hours to clear the system, then try a small sample and slowly increase the amount until a full serving is had. Once you are sure that you can digest both wheat and dairy separately, when keeping a nightshade free diet. Then try having wheat and dairy at the same time in small amounts. Until full serving sizes are achieved, if a success, then you did not have an allergy to wheat and dairy but could not properly digest them when your intestine was inflamed from nightshades!

Be sure to consult with your doctor before attempting any change in diet.

*"A diet that consists predominantly of rice leads to the use of opium, just as a diet that consists predominantly of potatoes leads to the use of liquor."*
- Friedrich Nietzsche (1844-1900), A mad German philosopher

The following are copies of MSDS (material safety data sheets) for potato dust. These MSDS are used for workers who will be handling the potato dust, when it is applied as a pesticide for crops. Please note, the use of potato dust for a pesticide is not a concern, in fact it may be one of the only good uses of potatoes. This has only been included to support the claim that potatoes contain toxins. This is not a call to ban potato dust as a pesticide, or find any fault with the companies that produce it. Some of the non-relevant sections have been removed from the MSDS, to aid the reading. Below are two MSDS's from different pesticide companies:

---

# SIGMA-ALDRICH

MATERIAL SAFETY DATA SHEET
Date Printed: 08/31/2006
Date Updated: 01/29/2006

Section 1 - Product and Company Information
Product Name **A-SOLANINE FROM POTATO SPROUTS**
Product Number S3757
Brand SIGMA
Company Sigma-Aldrich Canada, Ltd
Address 2149 Winston Park Drive
Oakville ON L6H 6J8 CA
Technical Phone: 9058299500
Fax: 9058299292
Emergency Phone: 800-424-9300
Section 2 - Composition/Information on Ingredient
Substance Name CAS # SARA 313
A-SOLANINE FROM POTATO SPROUTS 20562-02-1 No
Formula C45H73NO15
Synonyms Solanine *** alpha-Solanin * alpha-Solanine**
RTECS Number: WF0250000
Section 3 - Hazards Identification
EMERGENCY OVERVIEW
Harmful.

Harmful if swallowed.
Target organ(s): Nerves.
HMIS RATING
HEALTH: 1*
HEALTH: 1
FLAMMABILITY: 0
REACTIVITY: 0

Section 11 - Toxicological Information
ROUTE OF EXPOSURE
Skin Contact: May cause skin irritation.
Skin Absorption: May be harmful if absorbed
through the skin.
Inhalation: May be harmful if inhaled. Material
may be irritating to mucous membranes and upper
respiratory tract.
Ingestion: Harmful if swallowed.
TARGET ORGAN(S) OR SYSTEM(S)
Nerves.
SIGNS AND SYMPTOMS OF EXPOSURE
This material is a cholinesterase inhibitor. Other
symptoms include abdominal cramps, diarrhea, tight
chest, and miosis. Nausea, dizziness, and head-
ache.
TOXICITY DATA
Oral
Rat
590 mg/kg
LD50[244]
Intraperitoneal
Rat
67 MG/KG
LD50
Intraperitoneal
Mouse
32 MG/KG
LD50
Remarks: Lungs, Thorax, or Respiration:Dyspnea.
Gastrointestinal:Hypermotility, diarrhea. Periph-
eral Nerve and
Sensation:Flaccid paralysis without anesthesia
(usually neuromuscular blockage).

---

[244] LD50: Lethal Dose 50 percent of the time. Meaning a dose of that amount will kill
have of the selected subjects.

CHRONIC EXPOSURE - TERATOGEN[245]
Species: Rat
Dose: 40 MG/KG
Route of Application: Intraperitoneal
Exposure Time: (5-12D PREG)
Result: Specific Developmental Abnormalities:
Urogenital system.
Specific Developmental Abnormalities: Muscu-
loskeletal system.
Species: Rat
Dose: 40 MG/KG
Route of Application: Intraperitoneal
Exposure Time: (5-12D PREG)
Result: Affects on Embryo or Fetus: Fetotoxicity
(except death,
e.g., stunted fetus).
Species: Hamster
Dose: 200 MG/KG
Route of Application: Oral
Exposure Time: (8D PREG)
Result: Specific Developmental Abnormalities:
Central nervous system.
CHRONIC EXPOSURE - MUTAGEN
Species: Human
Dose: 66600 UG/L
Cell Type: fibroblast
Mutation test: Other mutation test systems
SIGMA - S3757 www.sigma-aldrich.com Page 4
Species: Mouse
Route: Intraperitoneal
Dose: 330 MG/KG
Exposure Time: 3D
Mutation test: Mutation in mammalian somatic
cells.
CHRONIC EXPOSURE - REPRODUCTIVE HAZARD
Species: Rat
Dose: 80 MG/KG
Route of Application: Intraperitoneal
Exposure Time: (5-12D PREG)
Result: Affects on Fertility: Post-implantation
mortality (e.g.,dead and/or resorbed implants per
total number of implants).

---

[245] Teratogen: An agent or factor which causes malformation of the developing embryo.

```
Species: Mouse
Dose: 100 MG/KG
Route of Application: Intraperitoneal
Exposure Time: (7-11D PREG)
Result: Affects on Fertility: Other measures of
fertility
Alkaloid salts, solid, n.o.s. [poisonous]

US Statements: Target organ(s): Nerves.
UNITED STATES REGULATORY INFORMATION
```

# Material Safety Data Sheet

**Catalog Number:** 158222
**Revision date:** 24-Apr-2006
## 1. IDENTIFICATION OF THE SUBSTANCE/PREPARATION AND COMPANY INFORMATION
**Catalog Number:** 158222
**Product name:** alpha-SOLANINE
**Synonyms:** Solanine; alpha-Solanin
**Supplier:**
MP Biomedicals, LLC
29525 Fountain Parkway
Solon, OH 44139
tel: 440-337-1200
**Emergency telephone number:** CHEMTREC: 1-800-424-9300 (1-703-527-3887)
## 2. COMPOSITION/INFORMATION ON INGREDIENTS
**Components CAS Number Weight % ACGIH Exposure Limits: OSHA Exposure Limits:**
alpha-SOLANINE 20562-02-1 90-100% None
## 3. HAZARDS IDENTIFICATION
**EMERGENCY OVERVIEW:** Harmful by inhalation, in contact with skin and if swallowed.
**Category of Danger:**
Harmful
**Principle routes of exposure:** Skin
**Inhalation:** Harmful by inhalation.
**Ingestion:** Harmful if swallowed.
**Skin contact:** Harmful in contact with skin.
**Eye contact:** Risk of serious damage to eyes

**Statements of hazard** HARMFUL IF SWALLOWED. MAY BE HARMFUL IF ABSORBED THROUGH SKIN OR INHALED.

**11. TOXICOLOGICAL INFORMATION**

**Product Information Acute toxicity**

**Components RTECS Number: Selected LD50s and LC50s**

alpha-SOLANINE WF0250000 Oral LD50 Rat : 590 mg/kg

**Chronic toxicity:** Chronic exposure may cause nausea and vomiting, higher exposure causes unconsciousness.

**Local affects:** Symptoms of overexposure may be headache, dizziness, tiredness, nausea and vomiting.

Specific affects: May include moderate to severe erythema (redness) and moderate edema (raisedskin), nausea, vomiting, headache.

*That venemous solanum, that deadly nightshade, that drives its cold poison into the understandings of men.* – 1652 John Smith Selected Discourses

# In Conclusion

It has been proven that nightshades contain dangerous glycol alkaloids. It has been proven that these glycol alkaloids are neurotoxins. It has been proven that these glycol alkaloids can have many harmful effects on human beings.

It has never been proven the glycol alkaloids contained in nightshades are harmless or safe for human consumption at any level. People who choose to eat nightshade plants should be alerted as to the dangers of these glycol alkaloids before they choose to ingest them. It is clear that the regulating bodies, entrusted with the responsibility of warning the public of the dangers that may be contained in foodstuffs, have failed to do adequate research and inform the public of what is common knowledge in the scientific community.

If you feel you are suffering from any of the troubles described in this book, it is quite easy and inexpensive to find out if nightshades are bothering you. All you have to do is remove them from your diet for a month or two, to see if your symptoms are alleviated. There is nothing to buy, no medicines to take, no treatments, no fancy machines, just a simple change in diet.

By adding a little more bread and rice to your diet, you can easily replace the nutrition that was once supplied by nightshade plants.

## Institutions and Lawyers

Most institutions use nightshades, whether it is military, school, rest home, hospital, or even prison. Tomato and potato are mainly used as staples in the daily diet, as these are very cheap and plentiful sources of nutrition. In light of the poisonous affects of nightshades, it seems more than reasonable that people in institutions not be *forced* to consume nightshades. Perfectly good sources of nutrition exist, such as wheat (breads and pastas), oats, millet, and rice. These are healthy and affordable.

None of the aforementioned contain any neurotoxins, thus they are unquestioned in their benefits as staples.

Institutions should either remove nightshades from their menu or offer alternatives when nightshades are served.

It may also be of great interest to leadership in such institutions and even athletics, to observe the health benefits gained. With fewer joint problems and increased oxygen uptake, from the elimination of nightshades in the diet of those in their care, be they soldiers, students, or seniors, an increase in overall performance will be a welcome delight to all. Especially welcome will be a decrease in the need for costly supplements as vitamins and sports drinks. *"Solanine (100 µM at pH 7.4) caused a 90% inhibition of active calcium transport in rat duodenum. The inhibition of active calcium transport was accompanied by a 40% decrease in oxygen consumption."*[246] Nightshades can cause red blood cell destruction in vitro[247].[248]

After all of the enormous legal battles over the ill effects of tobacco, and the great sums of money that exchanged hands, it would seem of great interest to institutions to cease the forced menus of nightshades, knowing that they contain poisons such as solanine, that build up over time.

Once some crazed lawyer decides that nightshades are the source of his client's problems, the amount of trouble he can cause will be unimaginable. Just a word of due warning, that the quicker institutions distance themselves from nightshades, the less future trouble they may have. "Caveat Vendere!" (*seller beware*).

Many myths about nightshades continue in present thinking. Many good sources will state that only the green parts of potatoes are contaminated with solanine, and that if you cut out the bad part the rest of the potato is safe; this has long been known to be false. One publication,

---

246 SOLANINE AND CHACONINE: First draft prepared by Dr T. Kuiper-Goodman and Dr P.S. Nawrot Bureau of Chemical Safety Health and Welfare Canada Ottawa, Ontario, Canada
247 Vitro: in glass, test tube or dish.
248 Kingsbury JM. Poisonous plants of the United States and Canada. New Jersey: Prentice-Hall, 1968; 288.

"Toxins A to Z, University of California Press," does not list solanine as a toxin, but it does list such things as caffeine. There is a problem with public knowledge, not with research; even respected institutions are failing to admit or announce that the toxins in nightshades exist. There needs to be a public education campaign of the health concerns regarding nightshades. Most every department of veterinary science will tell you quickly that livestock must not be allowed to eat nightshades; it is not a problem of knowledge, it is a problem of public knowledge.

*"Just put the potato down and nobody gets hurt"*

## Addicted to Spuds

Yes, with all of that nicotine and solanine in nightshades, you are addicted to spuds. Nicotine has been found to be one of hardest addictions to break. This is why most people "love" potatoes. It is for this reason that many think if you are trying to quit smoking, and are still eating nightshades, you are just making the whole process worse. It is advisable for someone who is trying to quit smoking, to also quit the other sources of nicotine, meaning those harmless looking taters on your plate. There you are trying to kick-the-habit and those little spuds, are stabbing you in the back with more nicotine–that just inflames your addiction.

# Nightshadefree.com

Please visit my web site at, www.taterhaters.com. I would love to hear from you, and would be glad to receive your stories of experience with nightshades for future work. We also have a forum available for people to discuss problems and solutions with nightshades, at the same address.

Email me at: michael@nightshadefree.com

Please join us at www.nightshadefree.com


**For book orders:**
>        sales@grassfiremedia.com
>        or
>        **www.grassfiremedia.com** for online orders


"You don't yet know the power of the nightshade!"
-Darth Tater

# Resources

Internet

- www.noarthritis.com
- www.nomato.com (tomato free ketchup)

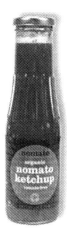

Organizations

- Arthritis Nightshades Research Foundation, 177 San Ramon Drive, San Jose, CA 95111-3615, USA.

## Title 17, U. S. Code

Notwithstanding the provisions of sections 106 and 106A, the fair use of a copyrighted work, including such use by reproduction in copies or phonorecords or by any other means specified by that section, for purposes such as criticism, comment, news reporting, teaching (including multiple copies for classroom use), scholarship, or research, is not an infringement of copyright. In determining whether the use made of a work in any particular case is a fair use the factors to be considered shall include—

- the purpose and character of the use, including whether such use is of a commercial nature or is for nonprofit educational purposes;
- the nature of the copyrighted work;
- the amount and substantiality of the portion used in relation to the copyrighted work as a whole; and
- the effect of the use upon the potential market for or value of the copyrighted work.

The fact that a work is unpublished shall not itself bar a finding of fair use if such finding is made upon consideration of all the above factors.

# Glossary

**(AChE) Acetylcholinesterase:** an enzyme that hydrolyzes (breaks down) acetylcholine in the synaptic cleft. Acetylcholine is involved in memory and learning. By inhibiting AChE, more acetylcholine becomes available to stimulate neurons, which can overwhelm the nervous system.

**(ACh) Acetylcholine:** is a neurotransmitter, liberated at nerve endings. It enables the transfer of information in the nervous system. It is important for forming memories, articulating thoughts, concentration, and physical movement. Was the first neurotransmitter to be identified in 1914 by Henry Hallett Dale for its actions on heart tissue. It was confirmed as a neurotransmitter by Otto Loewi who initially gave it the name vagusstoff because it was released from the vagus nerve. Both received the 1936 Nobel Prize in Physiology or Medicine for their work. It is a chemical transmitter in both the peripheral nervous system (PNS) and central nervous system (CNS) in many organisms including humans. Acetylcholine is the neurotransmitter in all autonomic ganglia.

**Alpha-chaconine or Alpha-solanine:** Two glycol alkaloids found in nightshades plants. *See Solanine*

**Alkaloid (glycol):** plant based chemicals that contain nitrogen. Many alkaloids possess potent pharmacologic effects. The alkaloids include cocaine, nicotine, solanine, chaconine, strychnine, piperine, caffeine, morphine, pilocarpine, atropine, methamphetamine, mescaline, ephedrine, and tryptamine.

**Alzheimer's disease:** is a condition where there is a relative shortage of acetylcholine, along with a mangling of neurons, so as to cause dysfunction of neurons.

**Atropine:** is commonly used to treat asthma, brachicardia (abnormal heartbeat), gastric ulcer treatment, hay fever, to slow the tremors caused by Parkinson's disease, and even by the United States government as an antidote for poisonous gas. Atropine that is manufactured synthetically can be utilized in surgery to stop fluids prior to surgery and is used in nasal decongestants.

**Cholinesterase inhibitor:** (or "anticholinesterase") suppresses the action of the enzyme. Because of its essential function, chemicals that interfere with the action of cholinesterase are potent neurotoxins, causing excessive salivation and eye watering in low doses, followed by muscle spasms and ultimately death (examples are some snake venoms, and the nerve gases sarin and VX). One counteracting medication is pralidoxime as is able to separate the enzyme from the attacking agent. Outside of biochemical warfare, anticholinesterases are also used in anesthesia or in the treatment of myasthenia gravis, glaucoma, and Alzheimer's disease. In addition, such compounds are used for killing insects in a range of products including sheep dip, organophosphate pesticides, and carbamate pesticides. In addition to acute poisoning as described above, a semi-acute poisoning characterized by strong mental disturbances can occur. In addition, prolonged exposure can cause birth defects.

**Hepatotoxic:** Injurious to the liver. Chemicals that cause liver damage are called hepatotoxins. It is a possible side effect of certain medications, but can also be caused by chemicals used in laboratories and industry, and natural chemicals, like microcystins. For example, acetaminophen (Tylenol) can be hepatotoxic. Solanine is considered a Hepatotoxic.

**Neurotransmitter:** a chemical (Acetylcholine, dopamine, epinephrine, or norepinephrine) that transmits information across the junction (synapse ) that separates one nerve cell (neuron) from another nerve cell or a muscle.

**Neurotoxin:** A chemical that interferes or prevents proper functioning of the nervous system, normally interfering with signal transmission. It is a toxin that acts specifically on nerve cells – neurons – usually by interacting with membrane proteins and ion channels. Many of the venoms and other toxins that organisms use in defense against vertebrates are neurotoxins. A common effect is paralysis, which sets in extremely rapidly. The venom of bees, scorpions, spiders, and snakes can contain many different toxins. Many neurotoxins act by affecting voltage-dependent ion channels. For example, tetrodotoxin and batrachotoxin affect sodium channels, maurotoxin, agitoxin, charybdotoxin, margatoxin, slotoxin, scyllatoxin and hefutoxin act on potassium channels, whereas calciseptine, taicatoxin and calcicludine act on calcium channels.

**Nightshade Plants (Solanaceae):** White Potato, "the common potato", tomato, eggplant, peppers( pimentos, paprika, cayenne, chili peppers, red, green, bell peppers), tobacco, mandrake, jimson weed (loco weed), Prickly Nightshade (Horse Nettle), atropine belladonna (Deadly Nightshade)

**Organophosphate:** (sometimes abbreviated OP) is the general name for esters of phosphoric acid and is one of the organophosphorus compounds. They can be found as part of insecticides, herbicides, and nerve gases, amongst others. Some less-toxic organophosphates can be used as solvents, plasticizers, and EP additives. Early pioneers in the field include Lassaigne (early 1800s) and Philip de Clermount (1854). Organophosphate pesticides (as well as Sarin and VX nerve gas) irreversibly inactivate acetylcholinesterase, which is essential to nerve function in insects, humans, and many other animals. Commonly used organophosphates have included *Parathion, Malathion, Methyl parathion, Chlorpyrifos, Diazinon, Phosmet, Azinphos methyl.*

**Potato (Solanum tuberosum):** The common white potato is a member of the nightshade family. Yams and sweet potatoes are not and do not contain Alkaloids. The common potato weighs 100g (small). Is a perennial plant of the Solanaceae, or nightshade, family, commonly grown for its starchy tuber. Potatoes are the world's most widely grown tuber crop, and the fourth largest crop in terms of fresh produce (after rice, wheat, and maize), but this ranking is inflated due to the high water content of fresh potatoes relative to that of other crops. The potato originated in southern Peru and is important to the culture of the Andes, where farmers grow many different varieties that have a remarkable diversity of colors and shapes.

**Scopolamine:** (skoh - pahl' - uh - meen), is derived from the belladonna plant, and acts as an anticholinergic (that is, it interferes with acetylcholine, a chemical that allows nerves to fire), preventing nerves from working properly. In large doses, it is extremely toxic, severely lowering the activity of nerves in the autonomic nervous system (the part of the nervous system that controls involuntary activity, like gland activity or cardiac muscle movement). In medicine, it is usually used in the form scopolamine hydrobromide. It can be used as a depressant of the central nervous system, though it can cause delirium in the presence of pain, mydriasis (pupillary dilation), and cycloplegia (paralysis of the eye muscles). When combined with morphine, it produces amnesia and a tranquilized state known as twilight sleep. Although originally used in obstetrics, it is now considered dangerous for that purpose. Sometimes side effects of scopolamine can be mistaken for symptoms of cancer because of the nausea and anisocoria associated with brain tumors. However, scopolamine induced anisocoria clears up usually within 3 days.

**Solanaceae: see (nightshades)** is a family of flowering plants, many of which are edible, while others are poisonous (some have both edible and toxic parts). The name of the family comes from the Latin Solanum "the nightshade plant," but the further etymology of that word is unclear; it has been suggested it originates from the Latin verb solari, meaning "to soothe."

**Solanine, (Alpha-solanine, or a-solanine):** glycoalkaloid poison found in species of the nightshade family. It can occur naturally in any part of the plant, including the leaves, fruit, and tubers. It is very toxic even in small quantities. Solanine has both fungicidal and pesticidal properties, and it is one of the plant's natural defenses. It is a non-water soluble chemical that is not destroyed by cooking. It can be reduced slightly by deep-frying at high temperatures, 470°F, but not completely. It is a stable, powerful cholinesterase inhibitor. Solanine can cause muscle pain and spasms, joint pain and swelling, gastrointestinal disturbances, anorexia, nausea, vomiting and feelings of nervousness.

**Synapse (sin´aps):** junction between various signal-transmitter cells, either between two neurons or between a neuron and a muscle or gland. It is a very small gap in-between neurons; when neurotransmitters are produced from one neuron, the neurotransmitters jump the gap, and are received by the other neuron, which will cause it to "fire." This "firing" will only happen once enough neurotransmitters have jumped the gap. The human brain contains a huge number of chemical synapses, with young children having about 1016 synapses (10,000 trillion). This number declines with age, stabilizing by adulthood. Estimates for an adult vary from 1015 to 5 × 1015 synapses (1,000 to 5,000 trillion).

The word "synapse" comes from "synaptein" which Sir Charles Scott Sherrington and his colleagues coined from the Greek "syn-" meaning "together" and "haptein" meaning "to clasp." Chemical synapses are not the only type of biological synapse: electrical and immunological synapses exist as well. Without a qualifier, however, "synapse" by itself most commonly refers to a chemical synapse.

**Teratogenicity:** The production of monsters or misshapen organisms, ie. Birth Defects

# References

1. American Cancer Society, Inc. (2003)
2. Armstrong, W.P. 2001. Wayne's Word: 9 May 2001. http://waynesword.palomar.edu/wayne.htm (12 June 2001)
3. Arthritis Nightshades Research Foundation
4. Atropine, Dr LM Pinto Pereiro, The University of the West Indies
5. Badowski P, Urbanek-Karlowska B. Solanine and chaconine: occurrence, properties, methods for determination. [Polish] Rocz Panstw Zakl Hig 1999;50(1):69-75.
6. Canada's Herb Specialists Goodwood, Ontario L0C 1A0, Canada Editor: Conrad Richter
7. Columbia Encyclopedia, sixth edition
8. David Rhodes, Department of Horticulture & Landscape Architecture, Purdue University
9. Declan Butler and Tony Reichhardt, Nature Volume 398:651, April 22, 1999
10. Douglas L. Holt, Ph.D. Chair - Food Science Program & State Extension Specialist for Food Safety, University of Missouri - Columbia, 122 Eckles Hall, Columbia, MO 65211-5410
11. EPA Journal - Fall 1994
12. Fackelmann, Kathy A.. "Food, drug, or poison? (toxic plants used by tribal cultures as food or medicine) (Cover Story)", Science News, May 15, 1993.
13. Fox News 2001 By Steven Milloy
14. George Ohsawa, Macrobiotics
15. Hans Ruesch, op.cit. 1992, p.65-66
16. Harvey MH, Morris BA, McMillan M, Marks V. Measurement of potato steroidal alkaloids in human serum and saliva by radioimmunoassay. Hum Toxicol 1985;4(5):503-12.
17. History of Potato, 2004 by Linda Stradley
18. History Magazine - The Impact of the Potato, Jeff Chapman
19. Induction of the cholesterol biosynthesis pathway in differentiated Caco-2 cells by the potato glycoalkaloid alpha-chaconine.Mandimika T, Baykus H, Poortman J, Garza C, Kuiper H, Peijnenburg A.RIKILT –

Institute of Food Safety, Wageningen University and Research Centre, P.O. Box 230, 6700 AE Wageningen, The Netherlands; Division of Nutritional Sciences, Cornell University, Ithaca, NY 14853, USA. 2007 Apr 27;

20. INHIBITION OF RAT CHOLINESTERASE ISOENZYMES IN VITRO AND IN VIVO BY THE POTATO ALKALOID, ɑ-CHACONINE1,2 SYDNEY O. ALOZIE, RAGHUBIR P. SHARMA, DATTAJIRAO K. SALUNKHE (1978) Journal of Food Biochemistry 2 (3), 259–276. doi:10.1111/j.1745-4514.1978.tb00621.x

21. Inhibition of Human Plasma and Serum Butyrylcholinesterase (EC 3.1.1.8) by a-Chaconine and a-Solanine1 H. N. NIGG,2 L. E. RAMOS, E. M. GRAHAM,3 J. STERLING,3 S. BROWN,3 AND J. A. CORNELL4 * University of Florida, I FAS, Citrus Research and Education Center, 700 Experiment Station Road. Lake Alfred. Florida 33850

22. John W. Kimball, Ph.D. Harvard

23. Journal of Neurological and Orthopedic Medical Surgery(1993)12:227-231, An Apparent Relation of Night-shades(Solanaceae)to Arthritis, N.F. Childers, Ph.D. and M.S. Margoles, M.D.

24. Kolbel CB, Singer MV, Mohle T, et al. Action of intravenous ethanol and atropine on the secretion of gastric acid, pancreatic enzymes and bile acids and the motility of the upper gastrointestinal tract in nonalcoholic humans. Pancreas 1986;1:211–8.

25. National Toxicology Program a -Chaconine [20562-03-2] and a -Solanine [20562-02-1] Review of Toxicological Literature, Prepared for Errol Zeiger, Ph.D. ,National Institute of Environmental Health Sciences

26. Orrego-Matte H, Fernandez O, Mena I. Affect of anticholinergic agents on the intestinal absorption of 59 Fe ferrous citrate. Am J Dig Dis 1971;16:789–95.

27. Organophosphate Insecticides Target the Serotonergic System in Developing Rat Brain Regions: Disparate Effects of Diazinon and Parathion at Doses Spanning the Threshold for Cholinesterase Inhibition

28. Theodore A. Slotkin,1,2 Charlotte A. Tate,1 Ian T. Ryde,1 Edward D. Levin,1,2 and Frederic J. Seidler

29. Poisonous Plants of Pennsylvania, Penn State, Veterinary Science Information, VSE 00-05

30. "Potatoes in uniform.", Utenkova, Yelena. Russian Life, November 1, 1997.

31. Potato glycoalkaloids adversely affect intestinal permeability and aggravate inflamma-tory bowel disease.Patel B, Schutte R, Sporns P, Doyle J, Jewel L, Fedorak RN. Division of Gastroenterology, Department of Medicine, University of Alberta, Edmonton, Alberta, Canada. 2002 Sep;8(5):340-6

32. Principles of Biology, Dr. Albert Harris, University of North Carolina, Chapel Hill

33. Qicheng F. Some current study and research approaches relating to the use of plants in the traditional Chinese medicine. J Ethnophar-macol 1980;2:57–63.

34. Robert Sharpe, op. cit. 1988, p.47

35. SOLANINE AND CHACONINE, Dr T. Kuiper-Goodman and Dr P.S. Nawrot Bureau of Chemical Safety Health and Welfare Canada Ottawa, Ontario, Canada

36. Solanine, Davey Stoker, Lincoln College, Oxford University.

37. Stephen Cooter, Ph.D. (Trees of Death)

38. Synergistic interaction of glycoalkaloids alpha-chaconine and alpha-solanine on developmental toxicity in Xenopus embryos.Rayburn- JR, Friedman M, Bantle JA.-US Environmental Protection Agency, Environmental Research Laboratory, Gulf Breeze, FL 32561, USA. 1995 Dec;33(12):1013-9.

39. Textbook of Military Medicine: Medical Aspects of Chemical and Biological Warfare: Chapter 5, Nerve Agents, Frederick R. Sidell, M.D

40. The Irish Potato Famine, by Catharina Japikse

41. History of Witchcraft, By Christina Hole, out of print

42. The Journal of the American Medical Association, March 24, 2000

43. The Potato-How the humble little spud rescued the western world. Larry Zuckerman,

44. THE SILENT WEAPON - Poisons and Antidotes in the Middle Ages by Gunnora Hallakarva.

45. University of Washington, Dr. Chudler

46. Webster's Medical Dictionary

47. Wikipedia

# Index

# Nightshade Survey

Included is a survey that you can use to see what effects nightshades have on you. First is a list of problems you now have. Carefully read over the list once without filling it out so you a general idea of the types of questions that are being asked, so as to avoid answer one question that sort of fit, compared to a latter question that fits better.

Then is a body chart for you to circle the areas which give you pain, be sure to mark each pain, even if you can stand it. Often we ignore pain, but in this survey we want a careful assessment of each and everyone.

Next is the calendar with the nightshades listed, if you eat nightshades on any certain day, mark them down by type and amount.

Last is the end of survey results, it is identical to the first inventory, because we want to see what pains or problems disappeared. This allows you to do your own experiment on yourself, rather than taking someone's word as to the effects of nightshades.

Included here are health assessment surveys, you may wish to fill them out on another piece of paper, or go to our website and fill out a survey that will give us valuable information in this cause of understanding nightshades.

## B1. Brief Pain Inventory (Short Form)

Date:____/____/____

1) Throughout our lives, most of us have had pain from time to time (such as minor headaches, sprains, and toothaches). Have you had pain other than these everyday kinds of pain today?     1. yes          2. no

2) On the diagram, mark in the areas where you feel pain. Use X for burning pain, N for stabbing pain, = for dull pain, and /// for numbness. Label each pain area with a number from 1-10 with 10 being the worst pain imagin-able, such as having your foot being run over by a car. You may wish to draw a line from the area of pain to the number.

*example*[249]

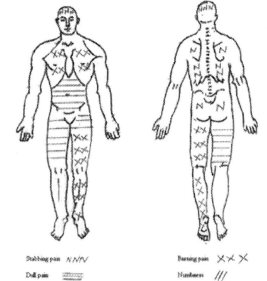

---

[249] Image courtesy: K.S. Ong and R.A. Seymour*
National University of Singapore, Faculty of Dentistry, Department of Oral and Maxillofacial Surgery, Singapore. *University of Newcastle-upon-Tyne, Faculty of Dentistry, Department of Restorative Dentistry, Newcastle, U.K.
http://www.rcsed.ac.uk/journal/svol2_1/20100003.html

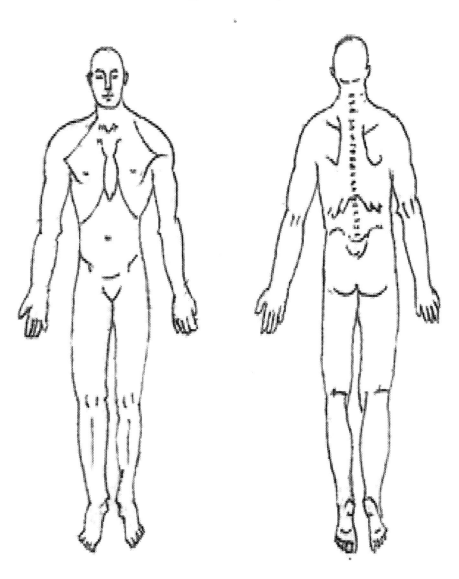

3) Please rate your pain by circling the one number that best describes your pain at its **WORST** in the past 24 hours.

| 0 | 1 | 2 | 3 | 4 | 5 | 6 | 7 | 8 | 9 | 10 |
|---|---|---|---|---|---|---|---|---|---|---|
| No pain | | | | | | | | Pain as bad as you can imagine | | |

4) Please rate your pain by circling the one number that best describes your pain at its **LEAST** in the past 24 hours.

| 0 | 1 | 2 | 3 | 4 | 5 | 6 | 7 | 8 | 9 | 10 |
|---|---|---|---|---|---|---|---|---|---|---|
| No pain | | | | | | | | Pain as bad as you can imagine | | |

5) Please rate your pain by circling the one number that best describes your pain on the **AVERAGE**.

| 0 | 1 | 2 | 3 | 4 | 5 | 6 | 7 | 8 | 9 | 10 |
|---|---|---|---|---|---|---|---|---|---|---|
| No pain | | | | | | | | Pain as bad as you can imagine | | |

6) Please rate your pain by circling the one number that tells how much pain you have **RIGHT NOW**.

| 0 | 1 | 2 | 3 | 4 | 5 | 6 | 7 | 8 | 9 | 10 |
|---|---|---|---|---|---|---|---|---|---|---|
| No pain | | | | | | | | Pain as bad as you can imagine | | |

7) What treatments or medications are you receiving for your pain?

8) In the past 24 hours, how much **RELIEF** have pain treatments or medications provided? Please circle the one percentage that most shows how much.

| 0% | 10% | 20% | 30% | 40% | 50% | 60% | 70% | 80% | 90% | 100% |
|---|---|---|---|---|---|---|---|---|---|---|
| No relief | | | | | | | | | Complete relief | |

9) Circle the one number that describes how, during the past 24 hours, **PAIN HAS INTERFERED** with your:

A. General Activity:

| 0 | 1 | 2 | 3 | 4 | 5 | 6 | 7 | 8 | 9 | 10 |
|---|---|---|---|---|---|---|---|---|---|----|
| Does not interfere | | | | | | | | | Completely interferes | |

B. Mood

| 0 | 1 | 2 | 3 | 4 | 5 | 6 | 7 | 8 | 9 | 10 |
|---|---|---|---|---|---|---|---|---|---|----|
| Does not interfere | | | | | | | | | Completely interferes | |

C. Walking ability

| 0 | 1 | 2 | 3 | 4 | 5 | 6 | 7 | 8 | 9 | 10 |
|---|---|---|---|---|---|---|---|---|---|----|
| Does not interfere | | | | | | | | | Completely interferes | |

D. Normal work (includes both work outside the home and housework)

| 0 | 1 | 2 | 3 | 4 | 5 | 6 | 7 | 8 | 9 | 10 |
|---|---|---|---|---|---|---|---|---|---|----|
| Does not interfere | | | | | | | | | Completely interferes | |

E. Relations with other people

| 0 | 1 | 2 | 3 | 4 | 5 | 6 | 7 | 8 | 9 | 10 |
|---|---|---|---|---|---|---|---|---|---|----|
| Does not interfere | | | | | | | | | Completely interferes | |

F. Sleep

| 0 | 1 | 2 | 3 | 4 | 5 | 6 | 7 | 8 | 9 | 10 |
|---|---|---|---|---|---|---|---|---|---|----|
| Does not interfere | | | | | | | | | Completely interferes | |

G. Enjoyment of life

| 0 | 1 | 2 | 3 | 4 | 5 | 6 | 7 | 8 | 9 | 10 |
|---|---|---|---|---|---|---|---|---|---|----|
| Does not interfere | | | | | | | | | Completely interferes | |

## Self-Assessment of Pain

Write any extra comments here in regards to pain only.

**Health Assessment**
Write out any non-pain related heath issues here.

## Nightshade Consumption Before Diet

Here is a chart to fill out the amount of nightshades you are currently consuming. Most people under-rate the amounts they eat, as they fail to included such things as tomato based pasta sauce, pizza sauces, salsas, green and red peppers, bell peppers, French fries, hash browns, mashed potatoes, etc. It is important to include foods that use nightshades as ingredients also. Many bread and dough manufactures use potato water to keep the bread soft for more than one day. Breads that stay soft for a week generally use potato water; it is not always clearly listed on the ingredients chart. Do the best you can to list all of the nightshades you eat and the amounts during a typical week. If the food includes nightshades then call it a nightshade-based food. Example: pizza is not tomatoes but it is a tomato-based food. A salad with a healthy amount of tomatoes is tomatoes–use your own judgment.

## Nightshade Consumption Chart

|  | Mon. | Tues. | Wed. | Thurs. | Fri. | Sat. | Sun. |
|---|---|---|---|---|---|---|---|
| Breakfast |  |  |  |  |  |  |  |
| Lunch |  |  |  |  |  |  |  |
| Dinner |  |  |  |  |  |  |  |
| Snacks |  |  |  |  |  |  |  |

# Notes

# Notes

# Notes

# About the Author

5 years old and 37 lbs, bleeding from the intestines and endless tests in hospitals; the very best in modern medicine was completely unable to help. No allergies were found; the little boy was suffering from malnourishment, even though there was food. It was as if his body was rejecting food.

Finally, by six years old his parents put him on a diet of chicken and rice. Only then did he start to thrive. The doctors said to introduce all other foods, that as he grew older he would adapt to the new foods. They were wrong.

This book should change the current thinking of modern medicine in regards to nightshade plants–at least that is the author's hope. If not, it should allow many people to self-cure. Somewhere out there are more little boy and girls, suffering from the toxic effects of nightshade plants. That is why this book was written.

The author was affected for years with severe cramping and intestinal disorders. He was misdiagnosed with Celiac's Disease. After eliminating wheat and dairy from his diet, as is the treatment, he still suffered from the original ailment. It was only by accident that a friend of his alerted him to the fact that potatoes contain solanine.

By eliminating potatoes, and other members of the nightshade family, he was for the first time able to lead a normal digestive life. Many joint problems dissipated, along with the severe intestinal cramping he had experienced over his whole life.

After much research and experiment, he was able to determine that this is a much larger problem than most people understand.

LaVergne, TN USA
05 November 2009
163167LV00009B/126/A